A FIELD GUIDE TO MEDICINAL PLANTS

BOOKS BY ARNOLD KROCHMAL

Hortica Practica
A Guide to Medicinal Plants of Appalachia
The Complete Illustrated Guide to Dyes from Natural Sources
Useful Plants of the Blue Ridge
Uncultivated Nuts of the United States
Gardening in the Carolinas
Indoor Gardening Green Thumb Guide
Let There Be Forest (with Connie Krochmal)

BOOKS BY CONNIE KROCHMAL

A Guide to Natural Cosmetics
A Naturalist's Guide to Cooking with Wild Plants
The Art of Wood Burning
A Walker's Guide to Nature
Caribbean Cooking *(with Arnold Krochmal)*
Making It—How to Do It for Less

A FIELD GUIDE TO
MEDICINAL PLANTS

Arnold and Connie Krochmal

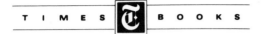
TIMES 𝕿 BOOKS

Library of Congress Cataloging in Publication Data

Krochmal, Arnold, 1919-
  A field guide to medicinal plants.

  Bibliography: p.
  Includes index.
  1. Medicinal plants—United States—Identification.
2. Materia medica, Vegetable—United States. I. Krochmal, Connie.   II. Title
QK99.U6K76   1984   581.6'34'0973   83-40321
ISBN 0-8129-6336-9

Manufactured in the United States of America

9 8

We are told by the Talmud that the world must have no fewer than thirty-six righteous men in each generation who are privileged to view the Divine Presence and who, by their acts and example, justify the continued existence of humanity.

This book is dedicated to the memory of one of those, a wise and loving teacher, a gentle and humble man, Dr. Walter Conrad Muenscher, Professor of Botany, Cornell University.

ACKNOWLEDGMENTS

We acknowledge our debt of gratitude to a number of people who encouraged and assisted us in this work.

First Ivan Dee, former vice-president of Quadrangle Books, who understood what we had in mind and wanted to do, and provided us with the opportunity and encouragement to complete the task. Our good friend Ted Larson, Prospect Park, Pennsylvania, whose support was essential to completion of the book; Julie Moore, Chapel Hill, North Carolina, who helped select a number of the plants included in our descriptions; John Reed, curator of the Library of the New York Botanical Garden; Dr. Earl Core, Professor, Department of Biology, West Virginia University; Dr. Frederick Meyer, curator of the herbarium of the National Arboretum of the United States; Dr. James Hardin, Professor, Department of Botany, North Carolina State University; Mary Ruth Chiles, Great Smoky Mountains National Park, Gatlinburg, Tennessee; Buford Muir, Chief of Photo Section, Forest Service, United States Department of Agriculture; Dr. Kenneth Muse, Department of Zoology, North Carolina State University; Christine Hopkins, Raleigh, North Carolina, and Mary Cowell, Photo Researcher, Office of Information, United States Department of Agriculture.

We owe special thanks to Dr. I. T. Littleton, director, D. H. Hill Library, North Carolina State University, Raleigh, who provided full support and cooperation by seeking out information sources enthusiastically and rapidly.

CONTENTS

A FIELD GUIDE TO MEDICINAL PLANTS

INTRODUCTION

Folklore and Science

We wrote this book for the increasing number of people who are concerned with the world of living things around us, particularly plants. We want to open the door on those plants that have been and still are used for the treatment of man's infirmities, mostly of the body but sometimes of the spirit. Through this work we hope to help concerned people learn that many a tree, shrub, or plant has served man's physical needs over countless generations so that they can recognize these old friends when they encounter them in the fields and forests. We hope to focus on the tremendous warehouse that nature provided for both our ancestors and us, a warehouse still awaiting the careful and scientific study that the twentieth century could provide but has done so, far too sparingly.

In the ten years that have passed since this book was first published, the use of herbs for healing has gained wider acceptance as well as respectability. In fact, in the early nineteen seventies herbal products were sold with a note on the package stating that the contents were dietary supplements. Now herbal products are sold with information on specific uses, and many pharmacies have available printed information for treating specific human ailments with herbal remedies. Magazines advertise herbal treatments, sometimes including recipes.

Both naturopathic healing and homeopathic healing have expanded greatly and are practiced with legal sanction in many states. In particular, the herbal tradition persists in any urban area where there are a substantial number of ethnic Chinese. The herbal dispenser may have as many as five hundred different herbal materials available for his clients, who come in a steady stream to continue the use of their traditional healing practices. A visit to any such locale in a large city will show a number of stores with herb displays in their windows, mostly imported medicinal plants from China, either in the dried botanical form or in packages.

Although great expansion has been made in the United States in the increased uses of herbal treatments, we lag behind other countries. In Moscow, where the two of us lectured on native American healing at the invitation of the Academy of the U.S.S.R., there is a prestigious Institute of Medicinal Plants devoted to research on the uses of such plants for healing man's diseases.

In Great Britain, Parliament has enacted legislation that has legitimized herbal healing and established internships for practitioners at teaching hospitals. Herbal materials used in Great Britain are analyzed for active ingredients so that proper dosages can be administered to the patient.

In India there are several Institutes devoted to the study of the cultivation of healing herbs, their uses and limitations, and their distribution in the forests of India.

In Romania, where we have spent two periods of study and research as guests of the Romanian Academy in an exchange program with the National Academy of Science, we found that pharmacies existed on three levels—the classical, including chemical and herbal materials; the homeopathic, which handled only plant remedies; and herbal sources, which sell traditional herbal materials in attractive packages.

We have lectured on herbal medicine at the Agricultural University at Wageningen, The Netherlands, and were able to visit a large herbal co-op whose members produce a variety of herbal plant materials, most of which are dispensed in homeopathic pharmacies, which are established all over Holland.

In India, generations of herbalists have used a plant, *Rauwolfia serpentina,* to calm the nerves of disturbed people. Only within the past twenty-five years has science shown that this plant is a reputable and useful source of a tranquilizing drug, rauwolfia, which is now marketed throughout the world.

Another example is ginseng, *Panax quinquefolius,* a plant that grows in the Orient and in the eastern part of the United States. Chinese pharmacopoeias and herbals have recommended powdered ginseng root for a range of medicinal purposes for at least 1,500 years. We have always had a deep respect for Chinese medicine and have felt that, if ginseng has withstood for so long the tests of time and Chinese medical practice, surely it must be of therapeutic value. Our faith has been rewarded in recent years by the publications of reputable and recognized research scientists working on the properties of this plant in Bulgaria, the U.S.S.R., and South Korea. Marked stimulatory effects have been found in the human brain after the use of ginseng. Powdered Korean and American ginseng can be found in most natural or organic food stores. Ginseng root is found in Chinese herbal shops.

Indian tobacco, *Lobelia inflata,* is another useful wild plant whose value has been especially recognized in the past ten years. This low-growing, purple-flowered annual is the source of an important alkaloid, lobeline, which is used in a number of anti-smoking preparations. The plants have been harvested in Appalachia for a long, long time and sold to pharmaceutical firms, but in recent years, the number of people who are willing to hunt for them in the forest has dwindled. Our research has shown how to cultivate these forest plants successfully, and this will make it possible for the people of Appalachia to grow this valuable medicinal plant at small cost in their backyards.

Another case is that of a very common plant, pokeweed, or *Phytolacca americana,* found in the eastern part of the United States. This vigorous perennial shrub can grow under the poorest of conditions—along fence rows and in old abandoned strip-mine areas, for example. For a long time it has been used in Appalachia in a number of ways. In the early spring, the young leaves are cooked as a green vegetable; in the summer and fall, the dark purplish berries are made into a wine and sometimes into pies. Research has shown that in some manner the fruit inhibits the division of body cells, a basic requirement for the treatment of tumors and cancer.

In Ethiopia, an English scientist saw women using the fruit of a local poke, rich in sudsy saponins, to wash their clothes in streams. He noted that near the laundry site there were large numbers of dead snails. This is interesting because sweet-water snails are the intermediate host for bilharzia, a serious tropical disease in humans. Although the Ethiopian poke is a different species from our native poke, the two are very closely related. Bilharzia exists in Puerto Rico.

A major step forward in recognizing the value of traditional healing methods, including herbal useage, came in 1981 with the opening of the Indian Service Hospital on the Cherokee reservation in North Carolina. It is a modern hospital with the latest and most advanced facilities and a staff of six physicians, three dentists, registered and practical nurses, and other medical professionals to provide care for members of the Cherokee nation. The crowning touch is the inclusion of a traditional healer whose office is exactly the same as those of the other medical professionals. Patients have the choice of using the services of the traditional healer or the classical medical practitioners.

Ironically, while medicinal plant use expands in the United States, and the world, funds for research have been substantially reduced at all levels. A twenty-five-year-old cooperative program in which the U.S. Department of Agriculture provided to the National Cancer Institute plant material to screen for anti-cancer potential was terminated in 1981. Dr. James Duke, chief of U.S.D.A.'s Economic Botany Laboratory in Beltsville, Maryland, calls this termination a ''...blot to natural-products chemistry in the United States.''

The work the two of us were doing in Kentucky with the cultivation of wild herbs that were used for healing (and were marketable as a means of providing cash income for the Appalachian people) regretfully ended.

More research, aimed at studying our own rich and varied flora for pharmaceutical use and at learning how to grow under cultivation wild plants that are highly marketable, would serve urgent needs. Such research would protect the more valuable plants from depletion. Crops requiring small capital input and small plots of land would provide rural people with a supplemental source of income and would give the pharmaceutical market a source of raw materials.

The Food and Agriculture Organization of the United Nations has pointed out that forests should be more than sources of timber for large corporations and an area in which urban dwellers seek recreation. The possible agricultural uses of our nation's forests are enormous, particularly those in the eastern United States, which provide the major portion of the wild medicinal plants that are harvested.

The people who live in and near forests, as do the people of Appalachia, are involved with the harvest of the forest understory plants for re-sale, a source of modest cash income. The management of the national forests should include information on the useable understory plants of the forest and their location.

Some Historical Background

As man became a settler and a grower of crops and animals, his knowledge of how to cultivate wild plants increased. Yet man has grown most of these plants for food and fiber, and only a small number for medical purposes.

We suspect that very early in his agricultural development man associated the wild plants he used for curative purposes with the untouched woods and forests. Perhaps he believed that these wild plants, because of their "purity" from man himself, were stronger and better able to fight diseases. To this day our sources of botanical drugs are plants growing in the wild—mainly in the forests of Appalachia, but also in the states along the Great Lakes and in the West.

Long before European settlers arrived on the shores of the New World, the highly developed Aztecs, Maya, Incas, and Indians of the United States had learned the medicinal uses of the plants growing around them. Some of these uses have stood the test of time; some have not. A huge number of plants await objective study to determine more fully their value for treating human ills (Figure 1). In South America, coca leaves were used by the Incas and the Aztecs to dull pain during surgery. Modern scientists have found that the leaves contain cocaine, which confirms the valid use of this plant by these early, highly advanced peoples.

An amazing number of plants used by the American Indians have been included in various formularies and pharmacopoeias in the United States and elsewhere, a

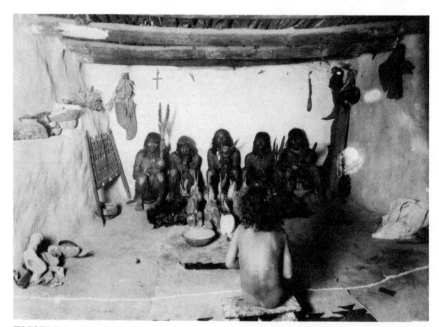

FIGURE 1. A sick Indian boy undergoing treatment by several medicine men in the Zia Pueblo, New Mexico, in the Kiva of the Giant Society.

tribute to the powers of observation and the medical skills of the first residents of the United States. For example, the Indians used club moss spores to help coagulate bleeding wounds and diminish scars. In 1960, the National Formulary listed club moss spores as a dusting powder for protecting tender skin surfaces. Indians used mayapple roots as a laxative, and, in 1950, the Dispensatory of the United States listed it for that use as well as others (Figure 2).

Indian healers used willow bark in a tea to cure fevers and colds. The active substance was salacylic acid, which the Germans synthesized after the Second World War to produce aspirin—to treat fevers and colds.

The Spanish settlers in the Southwest brought with them plant lore from Mexico, where their knowledge and experience with plants brought from Spain was augmented by the medicinal knowledge of the Aztecs they conquered. In the same way, the Moorish conquerors of much of Spain had earlier incorporated into Spanish herbal lore a great deal of the herbal lore of North Africa. African slaves in the South brought with them some of the same information brought to the new world by the Spanish. Thus the early use of botanical drugs in the United States was based on Spanish, Mexican, Aztec, Mayan, Incan, Indian, and African discoveries. The Spanish settlers, with the aid of the missions (Figure 3), both borrowed from and added to the rich store.

One of the favorite remedies of early settlers of the Southeastern states was yaupon, *Ilex vomitoria*. The Indians called a tea made of the leaves of this plant and another holly of the Southeast the "black drink." Along the coastal areas from North Carolina to Florida, it was drunk in the early spring both as a health measure

FIGURE 2. "Wu-nav-ai," a Paiute woman gathering seed of wild plants for herbal use in southern Nevada in 1872.

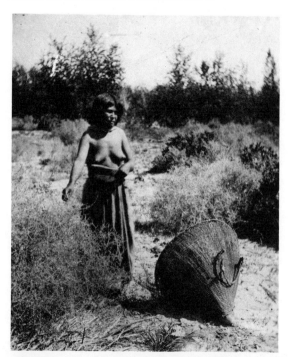

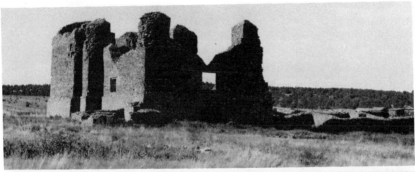

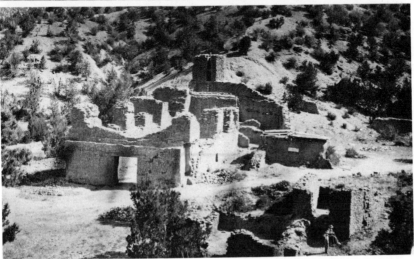

FIGURE 3. Remains of the Spanish colonization are to be seen to this day in the Southwest. With these churches as a center, information was gathered and ideas disseminated among the neighboring Indians, including the use of wild plants for curing sickness. Above, Laurel Mission near Punta de Agua, and below, Jemez Mission near Jemez, both in New Mexico.

and as a social activity (Figure 4). New Jersey tea, *Ceanothus americanus*, was a favorite tea substitute among the settlers during the American Revolution. They had noted that the Indians used it frequently. In Europe, research has shown that the plant has a potential for reducing high blood pressure.

Among the Indians, there were both medicine men and medicine women, although the men have been written about more often than the women (Figure 5). Today most Indian healers are men (Figure 6).

The fairly recent revival of interest in Finnish sauna baths recalls the Indians' use of hot baths for purifying the system and treating diseases. In underground saunas (Figure 7) or above-ground "sweat-lodges," heated rocks were sprinkled with water and often with aromatic plant parts. After using the sauna, the Indian men would dive into a nearby creek or stream.*

*"The sweat lodge was used for the curing of natural illnesses except for the common cold. The sweat bath was prescribed by both laymen and doctors to cure diseases. The heat was enough to induce an artificial fever which would aid recovery from some ailments." Harold Driver, *Indians of North America* (Chicago: University of Chicago Press, 1961).

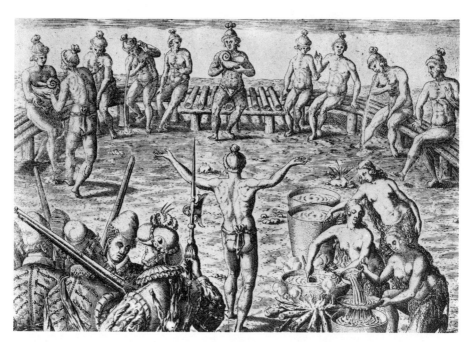

FIGURE 4. As part of a tribal ceremony Timuca Indians of Florida are shown drinking the "black drink" made from yaupon, *Ilex vomitoria*. One Indian is vomiting vigorously, part of the cleansing ceremony. (Sketch based on a drawing made in 1565.)

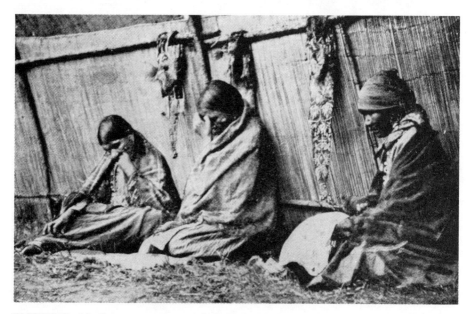

FIGURE 5. Medicine women were accepted and respected among the Indians. These medicine women of the Menominee tribe in Wisconsin are shown in a medicine lodge. (1925)

9

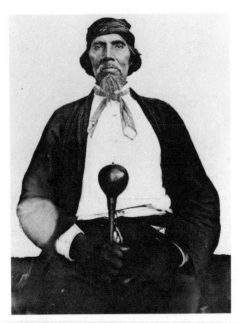

FIGURE 6. Swimmer, or "A'yun inĭ,"
a Cherokee medicine man. (1885)

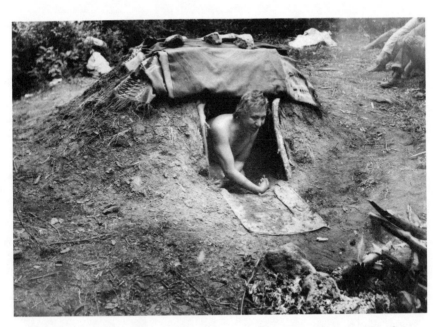

FIGURE 7. Underground sweat-houses, or saunas, were often used by the
Indians for purification ceremonies. This one was photographed in Washington
State (1937).

Hallucinogens

The hallucinogenic effect of certain plants was well known to the Indians, who used them to induce visions and transports, often as part of a religious ceremony. Despite this knowledge, the Indian users of these plants did not appear to become addicted.

Probably the most famous hallucinogen reported by Caucasians who observed Indian customs was the cactus peyote, or *Lophophora williamsii*. The buttons, or dried crowns, were chewed during religious ceremonies (Figure 8, 9, and 10), causing the participants to experience visions, hallucinations, and euphoria. The use of this plant is part of the ritual of the Native American Church. After some court action, this use has been accepted as legal for members of the church.

Another widely used hallucinogen was jimsonweed, a species of *Datura*. Various parts of the plant (roots, leaves, and flowers) were used to induce visions and bright colors, but on a less formal basis than peyote. Some young people have tried to "take trips" with jimsonweed seeds, sometimes with serious results. A friend of ours in Ohio reported that the police chief in his home town had found several acres of jimsonweed planted in a cornfield. We were asked if there was a market for the plant. Our answer was clear: "Not on the usual drug plant market."

Marijuana is not native to the United States, and so was not used by the Indians.

Plant Identification

To help identify the plants we discuss in this book, we have included very simple descriptions that emphasize the most visible and obvious characteristics of the plant. To round out these descriptions, we have included the best illustrations available. We hope that, between the two, the reader will be able to recognize the plants with relative ease. We have tried to illustrate all the plants for which a market exists, as well as those that have received a large share of early study and comment.

We have included as many common names as we could find, along with the scientific name of each plant. Common names are a source of confusion because almost every plant has a number of common names and because several different plants may share the same name. The common name at the top of each description is the one most widely used, according to a number of sources and our own experience. We have given first preference to the names recommended by the Subcommittee on Standardization of Common and Botanical Names of Weeds. Other sources were used where the committee had not made a recommendation.

Scientific names help in identification because they are generally recognized by most, if not all, botanists most of the time. Sometimes a name will change, but even an old scientific name will be useful in checking out a new one.

The Index of Plant Names at the back of the book should be helpful in tracking

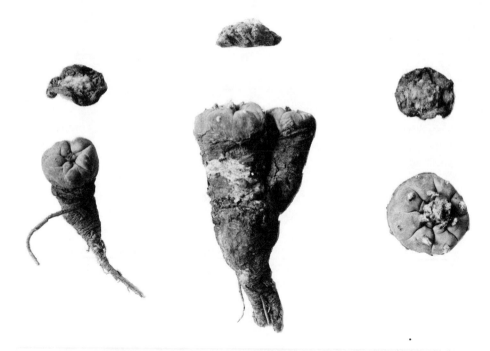

FIGURE 8. The dried crowns of peyote have been used by western Indians to induce visions and establish a feeling of well-being in religious ceremonies. The scientific name of the plant is *Lophophora williamsii*.

FIGURE 9. This is a photograph of "Many Tipi Poles" leading a peyote ceremony on the Kiowa Reservation in Oklahoma. He is holding a mescal rattle and staff. (1893)

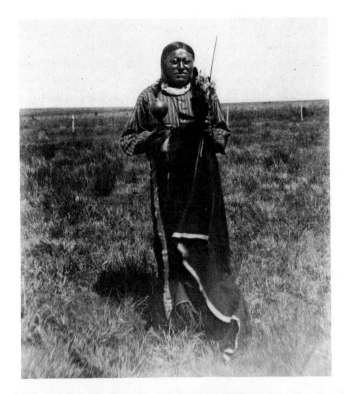

down plants. We have listed all names, common and scientific. Anyone knowing a common name should be able to look it up in the index and compare the description and illustrations with his own observations.

We have included a list of the ailments and problems for which the plants discussed have been used historically. THIS IS NOT MEANT TO BE A RECOMMENDATION. The variability in the content of plants' constituents and compounds makes casual use extremely dangerous.

We use the word *root* to describe any part of the plant growing below ground, although there are underground stems that outwardly seem to be roots, and roots occur in a wide range of shapes and forms.

We have used the term *bark* to describe the outer covering of woody plants. Any requirement for raw bark should be handled through sources we have listed. Cutting an entire ring of bark from around the trunk of a plant can cause serious damage and sometimes kill a plant or tree. Small pieces of bark are best harvested from limbs or branches. Inner bark is the material obtained by scraping the inside of bark. Root bark is found on the roots of some woody plants.

Preparation of plant drugs by use of water is variously described as making a tea, an infusion, or a decoction. The terms are not too distinct, and in old sources they overlap. Broadly speaking, a decoction is made by boiling a plant part in water. A brew may be the result of boiling the plant part in water or of allowing it to stand in hot or cold water. A tea is usually the result of putting a plant part into hot water that has boiled and allowing it to stand for five to ten minutes. An infusion results from keeping plant parts in hot or cold water for some longer period of time.

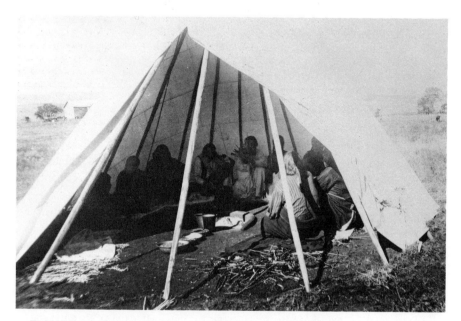

FIGURE 10. Looking into a mescal tent, scene of a peyote ceremony on the Kiowa Reservation in Oklahoma. (1893)

A poultice is hot or cold plant material, chopped and applied as a moist mass.

We have used the abbreviation *spp.* when several very similar species are used for the same purpose.

Drug Plant Sources

More than 85 percent of the medicinal plants harvested in the United States are found east of the Mississippi River, about 75 percent in Appalachian forests. Only a modest number come from cultivated sources. Probably the most important drug plant grown under cultivation in the United States is ginseng (*Panax quinquefolius* L.), which is cultivated in shade-houses in Kentucky, North Carolina, Tennessee, Michigan, and Illinois.

The collecting of wild medicinal plants has been affected by both social and economic problems. First, as rural people have moved from Appalachia to urban areas (about 20 percent of the population), Appalachian labor pools for plant collecting have been depleted. Second, as blue-collar job opportunities have increased and programs have been set in motion to provide gainful employment within Appalachia, the pressure to collect plants as a supplemental source of income has lessened. Third, in an era of "image" building, "toting a sack of yarbs" to a collecting point is not a job with a dignified image. Last, modern machine technology has entered the picture as well. Fifty years ago the market for white pine and wild cherry bark for cough remedies was met by hand harvesting. Now, sawmills supply large quantities of these barks as secondary products.

A very small part of our total need is imported. India sends us about $6,000,000 worth a year, Jamaica about $1,000,000 worth. Holland provides lobeline sulfate as an herb and in synthetic form. The total value of botanical drugs used annually in the United States is believed to be well over $500,000,000.

Synthetic Sources

In the United States, research goes on to find new drugs and to produce them synthetically. But the development of man-made substitutes for plant substances is not at all satisfactory. The time and costs involved in developing any new drug are astronomical, and, of course, these costs are passed on to the consumer. To justify such expenditures, a large and continuing market is needed. In many cases, the original source is cheaper and more readily available.

Then, too, some plants produce unique substances so complex that they defy synthesis, even in our era of great technological skill. Licorice root, *Glycyrrhiza glabra*, is a good example. We have imported licorice from the U.S.S.R., Iran, and Turkey.

Sometimes a wild plant can provide basic molecules that man can rearrange for his own needs. Such was the case with a true yam, *Dioscorea* species, growing in Mexico, where an American biochemist rearranged the molecules to produce cortisone. Now plantations of this yam are grown in Mexico and Guatemala by a German corporation to provide the raw materials for their cortisone production line.

Growing Drug Plants

Under some conditions, growing medicinal plants for the market is practical. A knowledge of what is marketable is important. The drug companies that buy such materials usually publish an annual list of what they want and the prices they will pay. We have included a list of some of these companies (see page 241).

A knowledge of which plants are adapted to your locality is necessary for success in growing plants, as is a knowledge of the germination and growth requirements for maximum yield. Unfortunately, such information is almost nonexistent for most plants. The mints, Indian tobacco, digitalis, ginseng, and basil are the principal plants for which some information is available. The others await study and research of the sort we did in Kentucky with wild Indian tobacco, mayapple, and poke while we were working for the U.S. Forest Service.

Annual plants are best for getting a cash return for the time, effort, and money invested. Those requiring two or more years are less attractive because of the delay in getting a return on capital invested.

Drying cultivated plants is not difficult. The basic requirements are a dry, shady area, preferably with some wind movement. The plants should not be piled too deep and should be turned carefully. Simple solar dryers can be used.

Caution!

Self-medication with wild plants is highly risky. Many of them are poisonous in the wild, unprocessed form. Plants harvested for commercial drug use are processed into something quite different before they are marketed. We urge and warn our readers to avoid using the information we have presented in this book to treat themselves for their own ailments. Much of the information about folk uses of medicinal plants is unproven by modern scientific methods, and some of the plants could kill you. In the summer of 1971, three young North Carolinians became violently ill after eating jimsonweed seed.

Arnold and Connie Krochmal

Asheville, North Carolina

September 1983

BIBLIOGRAPHY

Bailey, L. H. *Manual of Cultivated Plants.* Revised ed. New York, Macmillan, 1951.

Balls, Edward K. *Early Uses of California Plants.* Berkeley and Los Angeles, University of California Press, 1962.

Braubach, Charles. "Medicinal Plants of the Aztecs," *Journal of the American Pharmaceutical Association,* 1925, XIV, 498-505.

Burlage, Henry M. *Index of Plants of Texas with Reputed Medicinal and Poisonous Properties.* Austin, Texas, 1968.

Burns, Harold. *Drugs, Medicine and Man.* New York, Scribner's, 1962.

Clapp, A. *A Synopsis or Systematic Catalogue of the Medicinal Plants of the United States.* Philadelphia, T. K. and P. G. Collins, 1852.

Claus, Edward P., and Varro E. Tuler, Jr. *Pharmacognosy.* 5th ed. Philadelphia, Lea & Febiger, 1965.

Crawford, Howlette S., Clair L. Kucera, and John Ehrenreich. *Ozark Range and Wildlife Plants.* Agricultural Handbook No. 356. Washington, D.C., U.S. Department of Agriculture, 1969.

Curtin, L. S. M. *Healing Herbs of the Upper Rio Grande.* Laboratory of Anthropology, Sante Fe, N.M., 1947.

Darlington, William. *American Weeds and Useful Plants.* New York, A. O. Moore, 1859.

Dayton, William A. *Notes on Western Range Forbs.* Agricultural Handbook No. 161. Washington, D. C., U.S. Department of Agriculture, 1960.

Evans, J. R. "Medicinal Plants of the Cherokees." *American Pharmaceutical Association Proceedings,* 1859, VIII, 390-397.

Fernald, Merrit Lyndon. *Gray's Manual of Botany.* 8th ed. New York, American Book, 1950.

Fowells, H. A. *Silvics of Forest Trees of the United States.* Agricultural Handbook No. 271. Washington, D. C., U.S. Department of Agriculture, 1965.

Gilkey, Helen. *Handbook of Northwest Flowering Plants.* Portland, Ore., Metropolitan Press, 1961.

Gleason, Henry A. *The New Britton and Brown Illustrated Flora of the Northeastern United States and Adjacent Canada.* 3 vols. New York, New York Botanical Garden, 1952.

Gosselin, Raymond. "The Status of Natural Products in the American Pharmaceutical Market," *Lloydia,* 1962, XXIV (4), 241-243.

Grieve, M. *A Modern Herbal.* 2 vols. New York, Hafner, 1959.

Hardin, James W. *North Carolina Drug Plants of Commercial Value.* Bulletin No. 418. Raleigh, N.C., North Carolina State College Agricultural Experiment Station, 1964.

Harding, A. R. *Ginseng and Other Medicinal Plants.* Ohio, A. R. Harding, 1936.

Hayes, Doris W., and George A. Garrison. *Key to Important Woody Plants of Eastern Oregon and Washington.* Agricultural Handbook No. 148. Washington, D.C., U.S. Department of Agriculture, 1960.

Henkel, Alice. *Weeds Used in Medicine.* Farmers' Bulletin No. 188. Washington, D.C., U.S. Department of Agriculture, 1904.

Henkel, Alice. *Wild Medicinal Plants of the U.S.* Bulletin No. 89. Washington, D.C., U.S. Department of Agriculture, 1906.

Henkel, Alice. *American Root Drugs.* Bulletin No. 107. Washington, D.C., U.S. Department of Agriculture, 1907.

Henkel, Alice. *American Medicinal Barks.* Bulletin No. 139. Washington, D.C., U.S. Department of Agriculture, 1909.

Henkel, Alice. *American Medicinal Flowers, Fruits and Seeds.* Bulletin No. 26. Washington, D.C., U.S. Department of Agriculture, 1913.

Hocking, George. *A Dictionary of Terms of Pharmacognosy and Other Divisions of Economic Botany.* Springfield, Ill., Charles C. Thomas, Bannerstone House, 1955.

Imbesi, A. *Index Plantarum Quae in Omnium Popularum Pharmacopoeis Sunt.* Messina, Sicily, Adhuc Receptal, 1964.

Jacobs, Marion Lee, and Henry M. Burlage. *Index of Plants of North Carolina with Reputed Medicinal Uses.* Chapel Hill, N.C., University of North Carolina Press, 1958.

Johnson, Laurence. *A Manual of the Medical Botany of North America.* New York, William Wood, 1884.

Kearney, Thomas H., and Robert H. Pebbles. *Arizona Flora.* Berkeley and Los Angeles, University of California Press, 1960.

Kelsey, Harlan P., and William A. Dayton. *Standardized Plant Names.* 2nd ed. Harrisburg, Pa., J. Horace McFarland, 1942.

Krochmal, Arnold, and Sherman Paur. "Canai-
gre—A Desert Source of Tannin," *Economic
Botany,* 1951, V(4), 367-377.

Krochmal, A., S. Paur, and P. Duisberg. "Useful Native Plants in the American Deserts,"
Economic Botany, 1954, VIII(1), 3-20.

Krochmal, Arnold. "Medicinal Plants in Appalachia," *Economic Botany,* 1968, XXII(4),
332-337.

Krochmal, Arnold. "Deers Tongue, Trilisia
odoratissima: A Useful Plant of Southeastern United States," *Economic Botany,*
1969, XXIII(2), 185-186.

Krochmal, Arnold, and P. W. LeQuesne. *Pokeweed* (Phytolacca americana): *Possible
Source of a Molluscicide.* Forest Service
Research Paper NE-177, Upper Darby, Pa.,
1970.

Krochmal, Arnold, Leon Wilken, and Millie
Chien. *Lobeline Content of* Lobelia inflata:
*Structural, Environmental, and Develop-
mental Effects.* Forest Service, U.S. Department of Agriculture Research Paper NE-
178, Upper Darby, Pa., 1970.

Krochmal, Arnold, and Leon Wilken. *The
Culture of Indian Tobacco* (Lobelia inflata
L.). Forest Service, U.S. Department of
Agriculture Research Paper NE-181, Upper
Darby, Pa., 1970.

Krochmal, Arnold. *A Guide to Medicinal
Plants of Appalachia.* Agricultural Handbook No. 400. Washington, D.C., U.S. Department of Agriculture, 1971.

Little, Elbert L., Jr. *Check List of Native and
Naturalized Trees of the United States
(Including Alaska).* Agricultural Handbook
No. 41. Washington, D.C., U.S. Department
of Agriculture, 1953.

Massey, A. B. *Medicinal Plants.* Virginia Polytechnic Institute Bulletin No. 30. Blacks-
burg, Va., Virginia Polytechnic Institute,
1942.

Meyer, James F. *The Herbalist.* New York,
Rand McNally, 1960.

Miller, James F. *Weed Identification.* Athens,
Ga., University of Georgia Cooperative Extension Service, n.d.

Millspaugh, Charles F. *American Medicinal
Plants.* Philadelphia, Boericke & Tafel,
1887.

Osol, Arthur, and George Farrar. *The Dispensatory of the United States of America.* 24th
ed. 2 vols. Philadelphia, Lippincott, 1950.

Osol, Arthur, Robertson Pratt, and Mark D.
Altschule. *The United States Dispensatory.*
26th ed. Philadelphia, Lippincott, 1967.

Parker, Kittie F. *Arizona Ranch, Farm, and
Garden Weeds.* Circular 265. Tucson,
University of Arizona Extension Service,
1958.

Porcher, F. Pyre. *The Indigenous Medicinal
Plants of South Carolina.* Chicago, Trans-
actions of the American Medical Association, 1849.

Quer, P. Font. *Plantas Medicinales.* Barcelona,
Spain, Edit. Labor, S.A., 1962.

Radford, A. W., H. E. Ahles, and C. R. Bell.
*Guide to the Vascular Flora of the Caro-
linas.* Chapel Hill, N.C., University of North
Carolina Press, 1964.

Sargent, C. R. *Manual of the Trees of North
America.* 2 vols. New York, Dover, 1965.

Shelton, Ferne. *Pioneer Comforts and Kitchen
Remedies.* High Point, N.C., Hutcraft,
1965.

Strausbaugh, P. D., and Earl L. Core. *Flora of
West Virginia.* Morgantown, W. Va., West
Virginia University, 1952-1968. Published
in four parts as follows: Part I (1952), West
Virginia University Bulletin 52; Part II
(1953), Bulletin 53; Part III (1958), Bulletin 58; Part IV (1964), Bulletin 65 (with
introductory section).

Stuhr, Ernst T. *Medicinal Trees of the U.S.*
Portland, Maine, American Pharmaceutical
Association, 1931.

Subcommittee on Standardization of Common
and Botanical Names of Weeds. *Weeds.*
Urbana, Ill.: Weed Science Society of
America, 1966, XIV (4), 347-386.

Tehon, Oeo R. *The Drug Plants of Illinois.*
Illinois Natural History, Survey Circular 44,
1951.

Thornton, B. J., and L. W. Durrell. *Weeds of
Colorado.* Fort Collins, Col., Colorado State
College Experiment Station, 1941.

Todd, R. G., ed. *Extra Pharmacopoeia.* London,
England, Pharmaceutical Press, 1967.

Uphof, J. C. *Dictionary of Economic Plants.*
2d ed. New York, S-H Service Agency,
1968.

Vogel, Virgil J. *American Indian Medicine.*
Norman, Okla., University of Oklahoma
Press, 1970.

Watt, John Mitchell. *The Medicinal and Poisonous Plants of Southern and Eastern Africa.*
2d ed. Edinburgh and London, E. & S.
Livingstone Ltd., 1962.

Williams, Louis O. *Drug and Condiment Plants.*
Agricultural Handbook No. 172. Washington, D. C., U.S. Department of Agriculture,
1960.

GUIDE TO THE PLANTS

The medicinal, pharmaceutical or therapeutic uses of the plants discussed in this book are not to be taken in any way as a recommendation by the authors or the publisher. Some of the crude plant materials must be modified considerably before such use, and may be extremely poisonous when not used properly.

Readers of the book are cautioned against using these plant drugs for purposes of self-medication.

Abies balsamea (L.) Mill.

OTHER COMMON NAMES: balm of Gilead, balm of Gilead fir, balsam, blister pine, blisters, Canada balsam, eastern fir, fir balsam, fir pine, firtree, sapin, silver pine, single spruce.

PLANT DESCRIPTION: A tree, at maturity 40 to 60 feet in height, having a smooth, thin, brown bark, often with small blisters of resin. The twigs grow perpendicular to the branches. The needles are flattened, ½ to 1 inch long, dark green, and notched at the top.

WHERE IT GROWS: Low swampy areas, moist woods, near the timberlines in cooler climates. Minnesota, Wisconsin, Michigan, Iowa, the New England States, Pennsylvania, and New York to Virginia and West Virginia.

WHAT IS HARVESTED AND WHEN: Resin and needles, as needed; inner bark, during the growing season (but can be collected at any time).

USES: Indians rubbed the resin over burns, sores, and cuts and applied the same material to the chest or back to relieve pain in the heart and chest. The inner bark was made into a tea used to treat chest pains. Needles were placed on live coals in a sweat bath, and the fumes were inhaled for colds and coughs.

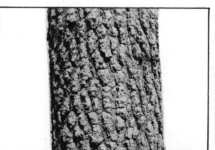

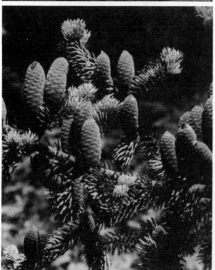

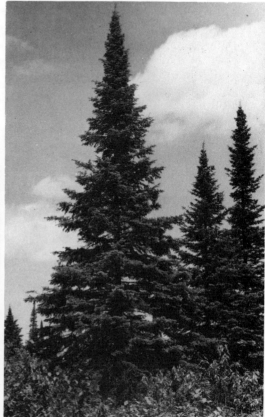

FRASER FIR 12

Abies fraseri (Pursh.) Poir.

OTHER COMMON NAMES: balsam, balsam fir, double fir balsam, double spruce, eastern fir, healing balsam, lashorn balsam, lashorn balsam spruce, mountain balsam, she balsam, she balsam fir, southern balsam fir, spruce.

WHERE IT GROWS: High mountains. West Virginia, Virginia, and Tennessee.

WHAT IS HARVESTED AND WHEN: Bark, as needed.

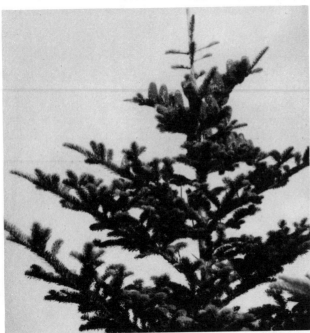

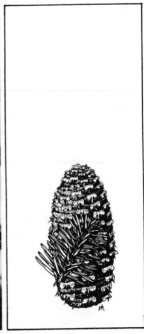

PLANT DESCRIPTION: A very resinous evergreen growing to 75 feet in height, with reddish bark. The needles are 1 inch long, shining dark green above, with two white bands beneath. The cones are 4 to 5 inches long, green to reddish brown.

USES: The bark has been used as a stimulant and to treat intestinal worms, clear the respiratory area of mucus, and increase urine flow. The turpentine has been used to aid in the healing of wounds and cuts.

RED MAPLE   13

Acer rubrum L.

OTHER COMMON NAMES: crable, erable, maple, red flower, scarlet maple, shoepeg maple, soft maple, swamp maple, water maple, white maple.

PLANT DESCRIPTION: A tree that grows to a height of 100 feet. The leaves are 2 to 4 inches long; the branches and flowers are red. The fruit is winged, ½ to ¾ inch long.

WHERE IT GROWS: Damp areas, along stream banks, and in wet swamps. New England south to Florida; Texas, Arkansas, Oklahoma, Iowa, Minnesota, and Wisconsin.

WHAT IS HARVESTED AND WHEN: Bark, as needed.

USES: Indians used the bark to make a decoction for treating eye ailments. The bark has been used as a treatment for worms, as a tonic, and in poultices for skin abrasions.

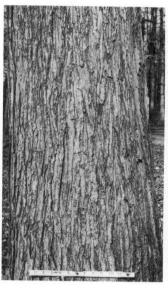
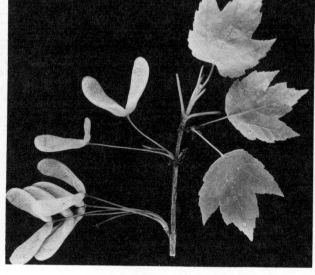

MOUNTAIN MAPLE 14

Acer spicatum Lam.

OTHER COMMON NAMES: goosefoot maple, low maple, mountain maple bush, spiked maple.

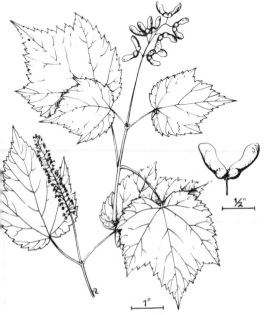

PLANT DESCRIPTION: A tree that grows to 30 feet in height. The bark is flaky or furrowed. The leaves are three- to five-lobed, fuzzy beneath, and have coarse-toothed margins. The small, greenish-yellow flowers are generally upright in spikes 3 to 5 inches long. The fruit is red or yellow, ¾ inch long.

WHERE IT GROWS: Moist, rocky hillsides, cool woods, usually in the shade of other trees. New England, New Jersey, Pennsylvania, Georgia, Tennessee, Ohio, Michigan, Wisconsin, Iowa.

WHAT IS HARVESTED AND WHEN: Bark, as needed.

USES: The bark has been used to treat intestinal worms, to stimulate the appetite, and to treat eye infections. In colonial times, a rose-tan dye was obtained from the bark.

COMMON YARROW 15

Achillea millefolium L.

OTHER COMMON NAMES: bloodwort, carpenter's grass, dog daisy, gordoloba, green arrow, milfoil, nosebleed, old man's pepper sanguinary, soldier's woundwort, thousand-leaf, thousand-leaved clover, thousand-seal, yarrow.

PLANT DESCRIPTION: A perennial that grows to 3 feet in height. The foliage is

lacy and graceful, the leaves aromatic. The stems are simple, without branches. The flowers are flattish and usually white, sometimes appearing purple, and are clustered in dense, flat heads at the top of the plant.

WHERE IT GROWS: Abundant in old pastures, fields, roadsides, waste places, and prairies. It is found in almost all parts of the United States.

WHAT IS HARVESTED AND WHEN:
Entire plant, in late summer when in full bloom.

USES: Indians used a tea made from the plant for weak and disordered stomachs. Colonists used the tea to break a sick person's fever by increasing perspiration, and to treat tuberculosis and headaches. The plant has been used as a tonic and stimulant, and to increase urine flow. A poultice made from the entire plant has been used to treat skin rash.

MONKS-HOOD   16

Aconitum columbianum Nutt.

OTHER COMMON NAME: Columbia monkshood.

PLANT DESCRIPTION: A perennial 1 to 5 feet in height. Its single stem, solid or pithy within, is more or less hairy. The flowers are purple to blue, with helmet-like petals about 1 inch long, usually beaked.

WHERE IT GROWS: Moist, shady spots along streams at elevations of 10,000 to 12,000 feet, in meadows, in deep rich soils. Oregon to Montana, south to New Mexico, Arizona, and California east of the Cascade Mountains.

WHAT IS HARVESTED AND WHEN:
Roots, as needed.

USES: The drug aconite has been used to treat pain from neuralgia, toothache, and sciatica.

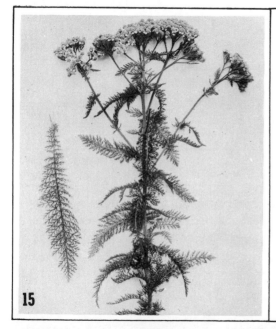

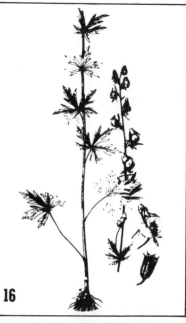

15

16

Acorus calamus L.

OTHER COMMON NAMES: beewort, bitter pepper root, calamus, drug sweet-flag, flagroot, myrtle flag, pine root, reed acorus, sweet cane, sweet cinnamon, sweet flagroot, sweet grass, sweet myrtle, sweet-root, sweet rush, sweet sedge, sweetsegg.

PLANT DESCRIPTION: A perennial 3 to 5 feet in height. The long, narrow leaves have sharp edges and are aromatic. The flower stalk, 2 to 3 inches long and club-like, appears about midway up the stalk. The flowers are greenish yellow.

WHERE IT GROWS: Swamps, edges of streams, and pond margins. It is widely distributed in the eastern United States, from New England west to Oregon and Montana, and from Texas east to Florida, and north.

WHAT IS HARVESTED AND WHEN: Rhizomes, in early spring or early fall.

USES: In Appalachia, the root is chewed to clear phlegm from the throat and to ease stomach gas. During a visit to Yugoslavia we learned that peasants use the root to induce abortion. An anthropologist friend tells us the same use is made of the **Acorus** in the highlands of New Guinea. Indians made an infusion of the root in boiling water and drank the fluid to treat pain in the stomach, gas, and stomach distress. The rhizomes have been used to treat coughs, flatulence, and indigestion, and have been considered useful as a tonic and stimulant.

BANEBERRY   18

Actaea arguta Nutt.

OTHER COMMON NAMES: chinaberry, cohosh, snakeberry.

PLANT DESCRIPTION: A perennial herb growing to 3 feet in height. The leaflets are 1 to 3 inches long, sharply indented, toothed, and egg-shaped. The flowers are small and white. The fruit is glossy, oval, white or red.

WHERE IT GROWS: Shady, moist places, on wet banks, along stream banks, beside springs, and in boggy places. Washington, Oregon, California, South Dakota, New Mexico, and Arizona.

WHAT IS HARVESTED AND WHEN: Seeds, in fall; roots, as needed.

USES: The roots have been considered laxative and capable of causing vomiting. They have been ground, mixed with tobacco or grease, and rubbed on the body to treat rheumatism. A pinch of the dried ground seeds added to a dish of food was once a treatment for diarrhea. Ground seeds mixed with pine pitch were applied as a poultice for neuralgia.

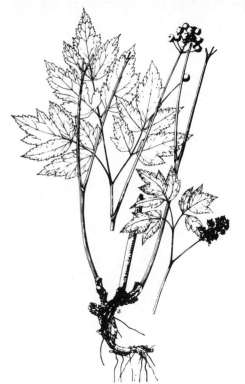

SOUTHERN MAIDENHAIR   19

Adiantum capillus-veneris L.

OTHER COMMON NAMES: black maiden's hair fern, lady's hair, maidenhair, true maidenfern, Venus' hair fern.

PLANT DESCRIPTION: A fern with small, stemmed leaflets arranged alternately along a stem. They are fan-shaped, pale green, with blunt edges. Their stems are deep red-brown to shiny black.

WHERE IT GROWS: Humus-rich woods, shaded areas, limestone rocks, and steep banks. Southeastern United States, including Virginia, Kentucky, and Florida, to Texas, Missouri, South Dakota, Colorado, Utah, and California.

WHAT IS HARVESTED AND WHEN: Roots and leaves, as needed.

USES: A tea of the plant has been used to treat coughs, respiratory ailments, and menstrual discomfort.

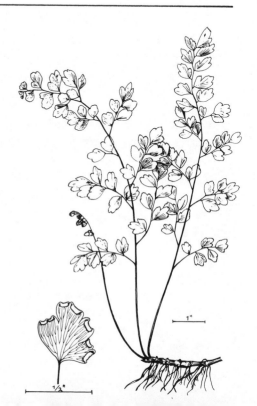

Adiantum pedatum L.

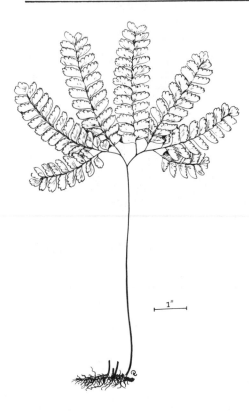

1"

OTHER COMMON NAMES: hair fern, maidenhair fern, rock fern, sweet fern.

PLANT DESCRIPTION: A fern with small leaflets arranged alternately along the stem. The stems are shiny black to deep red-brown.

WHERE IT GROWS: Shady, moist woods, steep limestone banks, and creek banks. New England to Minnesota, south to Oklahoma, Georgia, Alabama, Mississippi, and Lousiana.

WHAT IS HARVESTED AND WHEN: Rhizomes and leaves, as needed.

USES: A tea of the leaves has been used to treat coughs, colds, and hoarseness. The Indians used the roots as bitters and also for respiratory diseases. The rhizome has been used as a stimulant, to soothe the mucous membranes of the throat, and to loosen phlegm.

COMMON HORSECHESTNUT   21

Aesculus hippocastanum L.

OTHER COMMON NAMES: buckeye tree, horsechestnut.

PLANT DESCRIPTION: A tree that grows to 100 feet in height. The leaves have five- to seven-pointed leaflets, 4 to 8 inches long. The flowers have large white petals with red markings at the base, and occur in clusters up to 1 foot long. The fruit is round and prickly, and contains a shiny, round nut 2 inches in diameter.

WHERE IT GROWS: Slopes, wastelands, and woods. Georgia to Texas, north to North Carolina, Kentucky, and Missouri.

WHAT IS HARVESTED AND WHEN: Flowers, when in bloom; nuts, in late summer and early fall; bark, as required.

USES: In Appalachia, people have carried horsechestnuts in their pockets to prevent rheumatism. A tincture of the seeds has been used to treat hemorrhoids. An infusion of the bark or nuts has been used to cure skin sores and ulcers. The flowers have been used to treat rheumatism, the bark and fruit as a tonic and to treat fever. The fruit has been used to treat rectal complaints, hemorrhoids, rheumatism, and neuralgia.

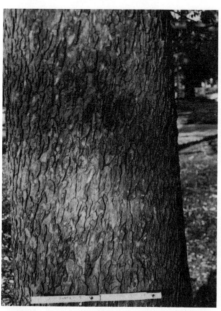

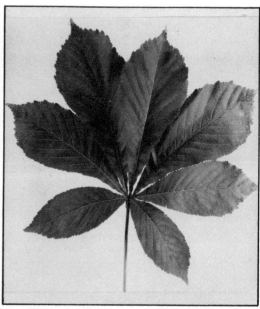

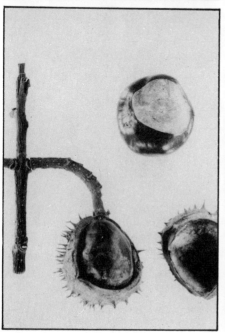

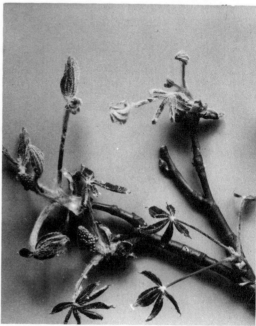

Ailanthus altissima (Mill.) Swingle

OTHER COMMON NAMES: ailanthus, Chinese sumach, copal tree, paradise tree, stinking chun.

PLANT DESCRIPTION: A tree that grows to 60 feet in height. The leaves are 1 to 3 feet long with many small leaflets, each with coarse teeth near base.

WHERE IT GROWS: Vacant lots, abandoned fields, open woodlands, and farm lots. All through the eastern portion of the United States and as far west as New Mexico and Arizona.

WHAT IS HARVESTED AND WHEN: Bark from trunk and roots, as needed.

USES: The powdered bark has been used to treat intestinal tapeworms and for

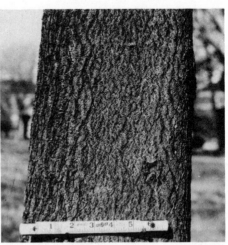

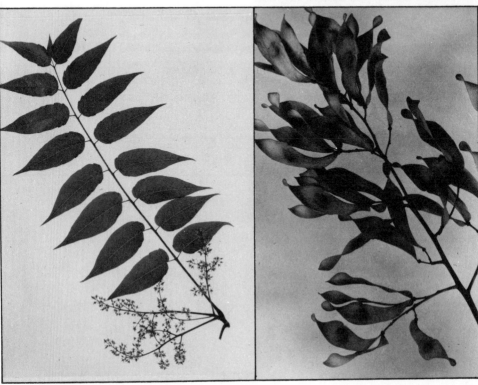

dysentery and other stomach troubles. The chewed bark causes cold sweats and dizziness. The root bark has been used to treat heart trouble, asthma, and epilepsy. In the early 1800's, the tree was believed to absorb malarial poisons. When malaria hit cities in which the tree had been planted, some people believed that the tree absorbed the poisons—but that it might also throw them off.

WHITETUBE STARGRASS 23

Aletris farinosa L.

OTHER COMMON NAMES: ague grass, ague horn, agueroot, aletris root, aloe, aloeroot, backache root, blazing star, colicroot, crow corn, devil's bit, false unicorn root, huskwood, huskwort, mealy starwort, rheumatism root, stargrass, starwort, true unicorn, true unicorn root, unicorn plant, unicorn root, unicorn's horns, white colicroot.

PLANT DESCRIPTION: A perennial with grasslike leaves in a flat rosette around a spikelike stem. The white to yellow tubular flowers are arranged along the stem.

WHERE IT GROWS: Moist locations in woods and meadows, dry or damp bogs. New England to Michigan and Wisconsin, south to Florida and west to Texas.

WHAT IS HARVESTED AND WHEN: Leaves, as they mature; roots, in the fall.

USES: In Appalachia, a mixture of roots and whiskey or brandy is drunk as a treatment for rheumatism. A poultice of the leaves has been used to treat sore breasts. The powdered leaves were once applied to sore backs. The roots were boiled and the liquid was drunk for stomach pains, as a tonic and sedative, and to increase urine flow.

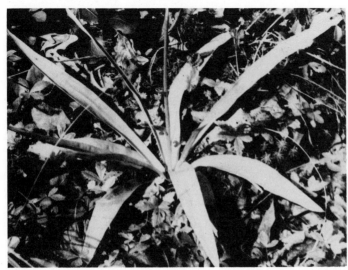
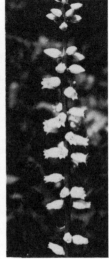

WILD ONION   24

Allium cernuum Roth.

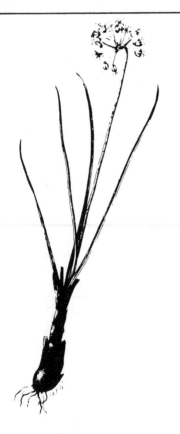

OTHER COMMON NAMES: nodding wild onion.

PLANT DESCRIPTION: A typical onion-resembling wild plant with pink or white flowers at the top and nodding to one side. Bulbs: 1 or more.

WHERE IT GROWS: In dry areas and at high altitudes. New York to Washington and Oregon and south to Tennessee, Georgia, Missouri, Texas, and the Plains states.

WHAT IS HARVESTED AND WHEN: Bulbs, usually in the second year or later when they are large enough.

USES: The uses of the wild onion and the garlic family are much the same. The bulbs have been used as a stimulant, to increase perspiration and urine flow, to expel intestinal worms, and as a cough remedy.

GARLIC   25

Allium sativum L.

PLANT DESCRIPTION: An annual that grows as high as 12 inches, arising from a bulb made up of several bulblets. The leaves are linear, long, and very narrow, arising from the base.

WHERE IT GROWS: Roadsides, pastures, fields, open woods, glades, and waste ground. Common in all parts of the United States.

WHAT IS HARVESTED AND WHEN:
Entire plant, when in flower; bulbs, in the fall.

USES: Garlic is the source of a compound called allicin, used to control worms in pets and people. A fresh poultice made of the mashed plant, applied three times daily, has been used to treat snakebite, hornet strings, and scorpion stings. The bulb has been browned in honey and butter and eaten to treat kidney and bladder troubles. To treat toothache, the bulb is pressed against the gum. Garlic has been eaten in food to expel intestinal worms. The fresh bulbs have been eaten to treat colds, coughs, hoarseness, and asthma.

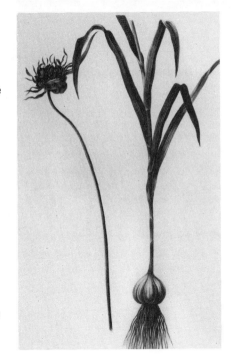

HAZEL ALDER 26

Alnus serrulata (Ait.) Willd.

OTHER COMMON NAMES: alder, American alder, black alder, candle alder, common alder, green alder, notch-leaved alder, red alder, smooth alder, speckled alder, swamp alder, tag alder.

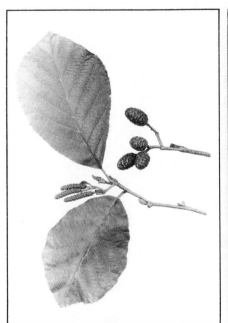

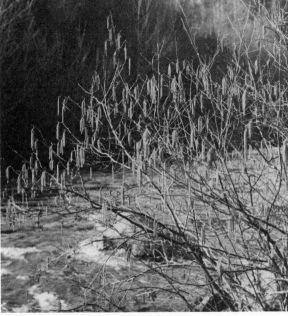

PLANT DESCRIPTION: A shrub or small tree growing to 25 feet in height. The bark is smooth and grayish, strongly aromatic. The leaves are leathery, 2 to 5 inches long, oval in shape, with small teeth around the margin. The flowers are borne in catkins; the female flowers turn woody and remain on the plant through the winter.

WHERE IT GROWS: Along stream edges, swamps, and coastal areas. New England to New York, Ohio, Indiana, Missouri, and Oklahoma, south to Florida and Texas.

WHAT IS HARVESTED AND WHEN: The bark of stems, in early spring or late fall.

USES: The dried, powdered bark steeped in water has been used for eye infections. In Appalachia, a poultice made of chewed bark is used to treat wounds and skin ulcers. Tea made from the bark has been used to treat diarrhea and as a blood purifier. A decoction of the bark was used in the 1800's to treat syphilis and malaria. A decoction of the catkins was a treatment for bloody urine. Indians applied an infusion of the inner bark to poison ivy rash.

SMOOTH PIGWEED   27

Amaranthus hybridus L.

OTHER COMMON NAMES: amaranth, careless, green amaranth, green opened amaranth, hybrid amaranthus, love lies bleeding, pigweed, prince's feather, red cockscomb, slender pigweed, slim amaranth, spleen amaranth, wild beet.

PLANT DESCRIPTION: An annual 1 to 6 feet in height, erect, branched above. The leaves are alternate, petioled, 3 to 6 inches long, dull green, rough, hairy, ovate, with wavy margins. The flowers are small with greenish or red terminal clusters. The taproot is long and fleshy, red or pink.

WHERE IT GROWS: Waste places, cultivated fields, barnyards, and orchards. Massachusetts to Michigan and Iowa; south to North Carolina; west to Texas, Arizona, New Mexico, and California.

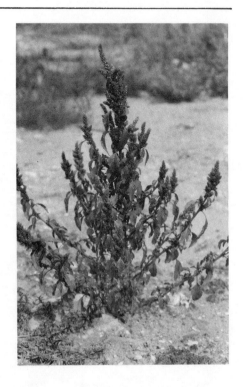

WHAT IS HARVESTED AND WHEN:
Leaves, during the growing season.

USES: The leaves are considered useful for reducing tissue swelling, and have a cleansing effect. The plant has been used to treat dysentery, diarrhea, excessive menstrual flow, ulcers, and intestinal hemorrhaging.

REDROOT PIGWEED   28

Amaranthus retroflexus L.

OTHER COMMON NAMES: beet-root, green amaranth, redroot, reflexed amaranthus, rough pigweed, tumble weed.

PLANT DESCRIPTION: A fuzzy weed up to 1 foot in height, with dull green leaves on long stalks. The flowers are densely packed in long spikes.

WHERE IT GROWS: Cultivated fields, lawns, waste places. Throughout the United States.

WHAT IS HARVESTED AND WHEN:
Leaves, from late spring into the fall.

USES: The leaves have been used in washing clothes because of their high saponin content. They have also been used to stop internal hemorrhaging, diarrhea, and excessive menstrual flow.

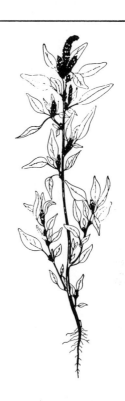

Ambrosia L. spp.

OTHER COMMON NAMES: feather geranium, giant ragweed, Jerusalem oak, Roman wormwood, western giant ragweed, western ragweed.

PLANT DESCRIPTION: A coarse, unattractive annual herb. The leaves are very dissected; the flowers green and inconspicuous.

WHERE IT GROWS: A wide range of sites in all parts of the United States.

WHAT IS HARVESTED AND WHEN: Entire plant, at full bloom.

USES: A poultice of the crushed plant has been used to treat poison sumac symptoms. It has been used to treat gonorrhea, diarrhea, and other intestinal disturbances. In Mexico, it is believed to be useful for treating intestinal worms and reducing fever.

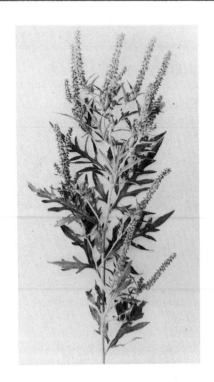

Angelica atropurpurea L.

OTHER COMMON NAMES: Alexanders, American angelica, angelica, archangel, Aunt Jerichos, bellyache root, common angelica, dead nettle, great angelica, high angelica, masterwort, masterwort aromatic.

PLANT DESCRIPTION: A shrub that grows to 8 feet in height. The stem is purplish with three toothed leaflets at the tip of each leaf stem. White or greenish flowers occur in clusters at the end of the stalk.

WHERE IT GROWS: Rich, low ground near streams and swamps, and in gardens. New England west to Ohio, Indiana, Illinois, and Wisconsin, south to Delaware, Maryland, West Virginia, and Kentucky.

WHAT IS HARVESTED AND WHEN: Roots, in the fall; seeds, when mature.

USES: Small amounts of the dried root or seeds have been used to treat stomach gas. In the 1800's, a doctor claimed that fifteen to twenty grains of the dried root taken internally would cause a revulsion against alcohol. The roots have been used to induce vomiting and perspiration; to treat bronchitis, rheumatism, gout, and fever; and to stimulate menstrual flow.

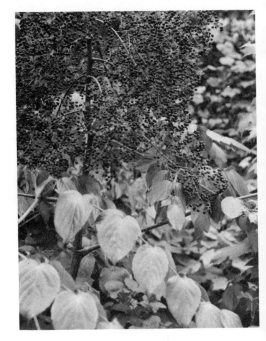

PUTTYROOT   31

Aplectrum hyemale (Muhl.) Torr.

OTHER COMMON NAME: Adam-and-Eve-root.

PLANT DESCRIPTION: A perennial orchid arising from a series of bulblike roots, with a single pointed leaf attached at the base. The flower, found on spikes, is purplish at the base, shading to brown at the top, with a white lip.

WHERE IT GROWS: Upland woods and mountains, shaded areas, and floodplains. New England south to Georgia, Tennessee, Kentucky, and Arkansas.

WHAT IS HARVESTED AND WHEN: The corm, in the fall.

USES: The corm has been used to treat bronchial illness.

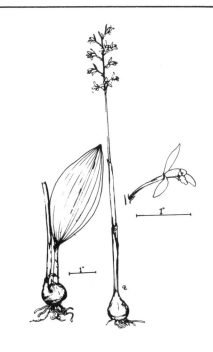

Apocynum androsaemifolium L.

OTHER COMMON NAMES: American ipecac, bitter dogbane, bitter-root, black Indian hemp, catch fly, colicroot, common dog's-bane, dogbane, fly trap, honey bloom, Indian hemp, milk ipecac, milkweed, rheumatism wood, wandering milkweed, western wallflower, wild ipecac.

PLANT DESCRIPTION: A perennial that grows to 6 feet in height. The leaves are opposite, the stems almost lacking. The flowers are oval, large, and whitish; the pods 4 to 6 inches long, and slender. The plant produces a milky sap.

WHERE IT GROWS: Along fences, borders of woods, old fields, meadows, thickets, and stream banks. New England to the uplands of North Carolina; West Virginia south to Georgia, Texas, Arkansas, New Mexico, and Arizona; north to Nebraska, Illinois, Indiana, and Ohio.

WHAT IS HARVESTED AND WHEN: Roots, in late fall; green fruit, in early spring.

USES: Indians believed that eating the boiled root would result in temporary sterility. The green fruit was boiled and used for a heart and kidney treatment, and a tea made of the root was used to keep the kidneys functioning properly during pregnancy. For headache, the dried roots were powdered and burned on live coals, and the fumes inhaled. A small dose of dried powdered root has been used to induce vomiting. The root has also been used to increase perspiration and as a tonic and laxative.

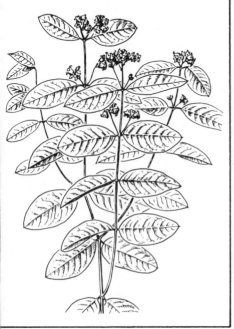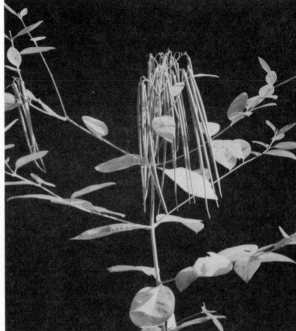

Apocynum cannabinum L.

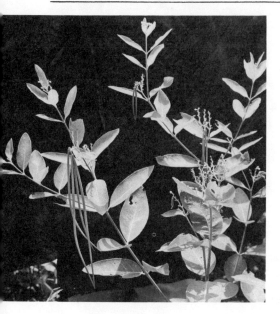

PLANT DESCRIPTION: A perennial growing to 6 feet in height, branched only at the top. The large, rounded leaves have short stalks. The whitish green flowers are borne on terminal clusters. The pods are double, 4 to 6 inches long, slender and pointed. The seeds are tufted. All plant parts produce a milky juice.

WHERE IT GROWS: Open ground, thickets, forest borders, and old fields. New England to Florida, Mississippi, Alabama, Louisiana, Texas, Arizona, New Mexico, and California.

WHAT IS HARVESTED AND WHEN: Roots and rhizomes, in the fall; entire plant, as needed.

USES: A half-ounce of crushed root was boiled in a pint of water and one or two ounces of the decoction administered several times a day as a laxative. The powdered root was used to induce vomiting. The entire plant, steeped in water, was used to treat intestinal worms, fever, dysentery, asthma, pneumonia, inflammation of the intestines, and indigestion. The plant is considered a heart stimulant.

OTHER COMMON NAMES: American hemp, amyroot, bitter-root, black Indian hemp, Bowman's root, Canadian hemp, choctaw root, glabrous hemp, Indian hemp, Indian physic, milkweed, rheumatism root, rheumatism weed, silkweed, wild cotton.

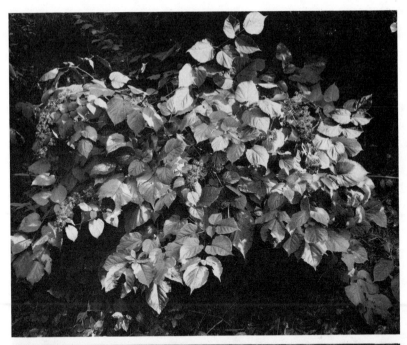

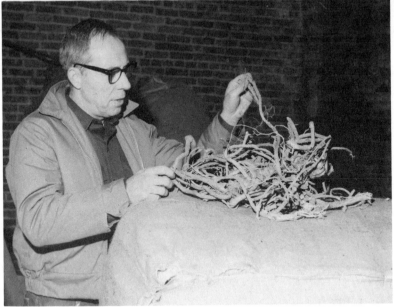

AMERICAN SPIKENARD   34

Aralia racemosa L.

OTHER COMMON NAMES: American sarsaparilla, Indian root, life-of-man, old man's root, petty morrel, pigeon weed, spignet, spikenard.

PLANT DESCRIPTION: A perennial 1 to 10 feet in height, with a single leaf stalk. The leaf is divided into three parts, each with five leaflets. The elongated flowering stalk bears yellowish green flowers in clusters, which produce a dark purplish berry.

WHERE IT GROWS: Rich woods, thickets, riverbanks and bluffs. New England south to Georgia, Alabama, Mississippi, Missouri, and Kansas.

WHAT IS HARVESTED AND WHEN: The roots, in summer and fall.

USES: The Indians made a tea of the roots to treat backache, and used a poultice made of the ground root to treat sores and inflammations. In Appalachia, a root tea is used to treat backache. The rhizomes have been used to treat colds, coughs, gout, skin diseases, and as a stimulant to increase perspiration and cure asthma and blood poisoning.

HERCULES CLUB   35

Aralia spinosa L.

OTHER COMMON NAMES: angelica tree, devil's walking stick, prickly-ash, prickly elder, thorny ash, toothache bush.

PLANT DESCRIPTION: A shrub or tree growing to 30 feet in height, with spines on the leaf stalks. The leaflets are toothed; the flowers white, and very small.

WHERE IT GROWS: Woods, thickets, and along fence rows. Eastern United States to Florida and west to Texas.

WHAT IS HARVESTED AND WHEN: Bark, as needed; roots, in the fall.

USES: Indians drank a decoction of the bark and root to purify the blood and to

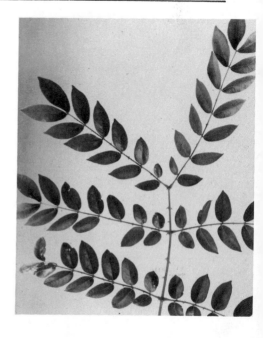

treat fever. They used the boiled mashed root as a poultice to bring boils to a head. Negroes used the fresh root to treat snakebite, and applied a dried powder of the root to the site of the bite. The water that fresh roots were stored in has been used to treat irritated eyes. The bark has been considered a stimulant and also a means of breaking fever by increasing perspiration.

GREAT BURDOCK 36

Arctium lappa L.

OTHER COMMON NAMES: beggar's buttons, burdock, burrseed, clotbur, cockle-button, cuckoo button, harebur, hare-lock, lappa, turkey-bur.

PLANT DESCRIPTION: A biennial or perennial 2 to 8 feet in height, with a many-flowered head. The leaves are large, broad, and rounded, like rhubarb leaves. The tubular flowers are pale pink, purple, or white. Big, round, brown, bristly burrs are produced.

WHERE IT GROWS: Waste places, roadsides, and abandoned fields. New England, New York, and Pennsylvania, and west to Michigan.

WHAT IS HARVESTED AND WHEN: Roots of the first year's growth, as needed; seeds, as they mature.

USES: In Appalachia, a tea of roots or seeds is used to treat rheumatism and to purify the blood in early spring. Powdered seeds have been used to treat sties and to increase urination. A decoction of the root was once used to treat catarrh, rheumatism, and gout. A decoction of the root boiled in water was used to treat impetigo. The squeezed leaves produce a juice that has been used for eye irritations. Pioneers used the plants to treat gonorrhea, syphilis, gout, and cancer. A cooling poultice has been made from the leaves and applied to skin burns and ulcers.

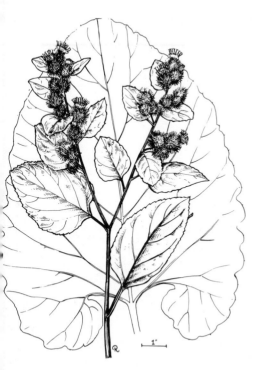

COMMON BURDOCK   37

Arctium minus (Hill) Bernh.

OTHER COMMON NAMES: burdock, clotbur, cuckoo button, lesser burdock, smaller burdock.

PLANT DESCRIPTION: A biennial or perennial 5 to 8 feet in height, with large, broad leaves resembling rhubarb. The tube-shaped white and pink-to-purple flowers are borne in many-flowered heads. Big, brown, bristly burrs bear the seeds.

WHERE IT GROWS: Wastelands, fields, and pastures. All parts of the United States from New England to California.

WHAT IS HARVESTED AND WHEN: Roots, in the fall of first year's growth; seeds, when they appear, usually in the second year.

USES: A tea made from the leaves or roots has been used to treat coughs, asthma, and lung disease and to stimulate menstruation. A tincture of the fresh root is also used for rheumatism and stomachache.

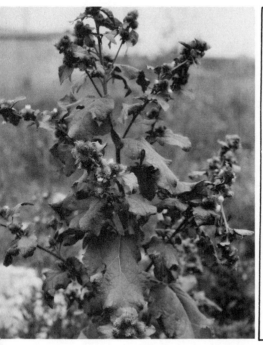
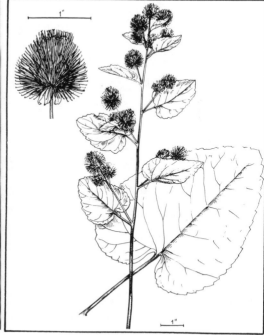

BEARBERRY 38

Arctostaphylos uva-ursi (L.) Spreng.

OTHER COMMON NAMES: arberry, bear's grape, coralillo, hog cranberry, kinnikinnick, manzanita, mealberry, upland cranberry, uva-ursi.

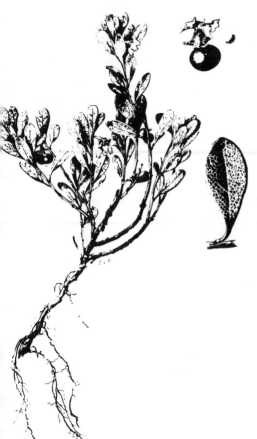

PLANT DESCRIPTION: A creeping evergreen shrub with stems up to 6 inches in height. The bark is reddish; the leaves bright green, 1 inch long; the flowers white with red markings, in clusters.

WHERE IT GROWS: Dry, well-drained soils at higher altitudes in conifer forests. From Oregon, Washington, and California to Colorado and New Mexico.

WHAT IS HARVESTED AND WHEN: Plant parts, in bloom; leaves, when mature.

USES: The powdered leaves were used to treat urinary problems. It was believed that they would help uterine contractions and aid in cases of urinary incontinency. The plant has been used to treat hemorrhaging, bronchitis, and diarrhea. It has been boiled and the infusion drunk for sprains, stomach pains, and urinary troubles. Indians mixed the dried leaves with tobacco and smoked the mixture. Pioneers in the West made a decoction of the leaves and applied it to poison oak inflammations.

INDIAN JACK-IN-THE-PULPIT 39

Arisaema triphyllum (L.) Schott.

OTHER COMMON NAMES: bog onion, brown dragon, cuckoo plant, devil's ear, dragon root, dragon turnip, Indian turnip, jack-in-the-pulpit, lords and ladies, marsh turnip, meadow turnip, memory root, pepper turnip, priest's pintle, small jack-in-the-pulpit, starchwort, swamp turnip, thrice-leaved arum, wake-robin, wild pepper, wild turnip.

PLANT DESCRIPTION: A small perennial with two stalks of three leaves each and a third stalk topped with a green tubular "pulpit" and a covering hood turned down over the pulpit. In the fall, the pulpit stalk has dense clusters of vivid scarlet berries.

WHERE IT GROWS: Swamps, bogs, and damp woodlands. New York, Massachusetts, and Connecticut south to Georgia and Kentucky and on the coastal plains and piedmont.

WHAT IS HARVESTED AND WHEN: The root, in spring or fall, plant, as needed.

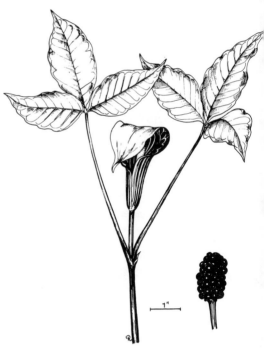

USES: The corms have been grated and boiled in milk and the concoction used to treat coughs and tuberculosis. Indians recognized that heating or drying the caustic fresh corms made them highly palatable, and they ate large quantities as food. The corm has been considered useful for treating stomach gas, asthma, and rheumatism. The plant has been used as an expectorant, as a skin irritant to cause blistering, and as a means of increasing urine flow. Some reports say that the root has been considered insecticidal.

VIRGINIA SNAKEROOT 40

Aristolochia serpentaria L.

OTHER COMMON NAMES: birthwort, Dutchman's pipe, pelican flower, sangrel, sangrel-root, serpentaria, serpentary root, snakeroot, snakeweed, thick birthwort.

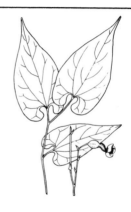

PLANT DESCRIPTION: This perennial grows to 2 feet in height. It has an erect stem and heart-shaped leaves that come to a point. Brownish flowers rise from the base of the stem.

WHERE IT GROWS: Rich woods, forests, and woodlands. Florida west to Texas, north to Connecticut, New York, Ohio, Indiana, Illinois, Missouri, and Kansas.

WHAT IS HARVESTED AND WHEN: Roots, in the fall.

USES: The earliest use of this plant was based on the belief that it could protect a person from poisoning. The finely powdered root was combined with white wine (1 part root to 3 parts wine) and used to induce sweating in the treatment of malaria. The root was also used to treat typhus fever, smallpox, and pneumonia, and applied as a poultice on open wounds and skin ulcers.

BIG SAGEBRUSH   41

Artemisia tridentata Nutt.

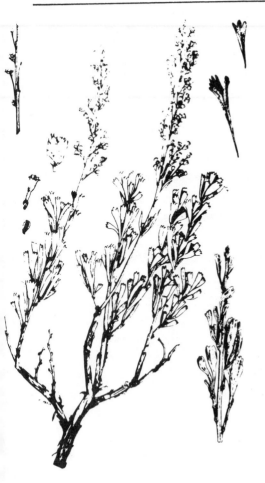

OTHER COMMON NAMES: basin sagebrush, chamiso hediondo, sagebrush, toothed sagebrush, wormwood.

PLANT DESCRIPTION: A shrub growing to 12 feet in height, much branched, covered with silvery fuzz. The flowers are yellow or whitish, in densely packed heads. The foliage is aromatic.

WHERE IT GROWS: Dry and sandy soils, on ranges and hillsides. Oregon, Washington, California, Colorado, Nebraska, and Utah. Reported in New England.

WHAT IS HARVESTED AND WHEN: Leaves and branches, as needed.

USES: A tea made of the leaves has been used to treat headache, stomachache, vomiting, diarrhea, sore throat, and as an antidote for poisoning. Some Indians chewed the leaves to ease stomach gas. A wash made of boiled and steeped leaves was used for treating bullet wounds and cuts, to bathe newborn babies, and as a hot poultice in treating rheumatism. A poultice was also placed on the stomach

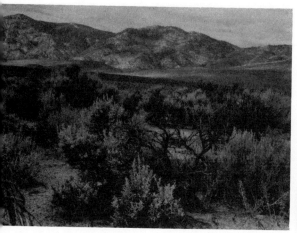
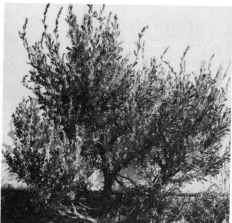

to induce menstruation, to relieve colic, and treat worms. The branches were often burned to purify the air in a room where a woman had given birth to a child.

CANADA WILD GINGER 42

Asarum canadense L.

OTHER COMMON NAMES: black snake-root, black snakeweed, broad-leaved sara-bacca, Canada snakeroot, catfoot, colic-root, coltsfoot, coltsfoot snakeroot, false colt's foot, heart snakeroot, Indian ginger, southern snakeroot, Vermont snakeroot, wild ginger.

PLANT DESCRIPTION: A low-growing, stemless perennial with heart-shaped leaves. Brown, bell-shaped flowers, purple inside, are found near the root. The stem has a spicy odor.

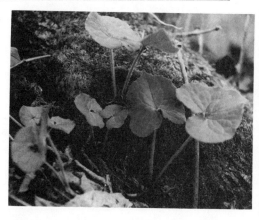

WHERE IT GROWS: Shaded calcareous ledges and cool, shaded, moist woods and slopes. New England, Appalachia, and along the coast states to North Carolina.

WHAT IS HARVESTED AND WHEN: The roots, at any time; the leaves, as needed.

USES: In Appalachia, a tea made of the roots is used to relieve stomach gas. The powdered root has been used to relieve gas and to induce perspiration. A fine powder of the dried root was inhaled like snuff to relieve aching head and eyes. The pioneers used the root as a stimulant and for heart palpitations, fevers, and nervous problems.

Asclepias speciosa Torr.

PLANT DESCRIPTION: A perennial with milky juice, growing to 5 feet in height. The whole plant is often covered with a short fuzz. The leaves are heart-shaped, the flowers purple.

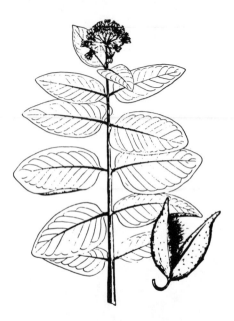

WHERE IT GROWS: Prairies and other sunny open areas. Minnesota to the Pacific Coast, south to Arizona, New Mexico, Texas, Oklahoma, and Missouri.

WHAT IS HARVESTED AND WHEN: Latex (juice), when the plant is mature and large enough to make harvesting worthwhile; entire plant in bloom or in seed; the roots of plants older than one year, in the spring.

USES: The milky latex has been used as an antiseptic for treating ringworm, cuts, and sores and to remove corns and calluses. After the seeds have been boiled in water, the victim of a rattlesnake bite bathes in the water. A tea made of boiled roots has been used to treat measles, coughs, and tuberculosis, and has been applied warm to rheumatic joints. The mashed roots have been used as a poultice to reduce swellings. Indian women used an infusion of the entire plant to treat sore breasts.

COMMON MILKWEED   44

Asclepias syriaca L.

OTHER COMMON NAMES: common silkweed, cottonweed, milkweed, silkweed, silky swallow-wort, Virginia silk, Virginia swallow-wort, wild cotton.

PLANT DESCRIPTION: A perennial that grows to 5 feet in height. Its leaves are broadly oval, opposite or in whorls,

fuzzy below, 4 to 8 inches long. The dull greenish purple flowers form a head.

WHERE IT GROWS: Thickets, meadows, roadsides, fields, orchards, and the edges of fields. New England south to Georgia and Tennessee and west to Iowa and Kansas.

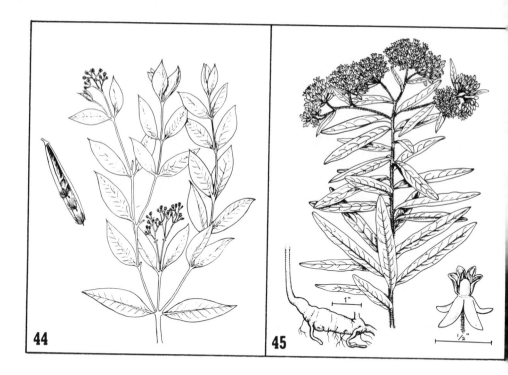

44 45

WHAT IS HARVESTED AND WHEN:
Roots, in the fall.

USES: In Appalachia, the milky sap is used to treat warts and moles. A decoc- tion of the root has been used as a treat- ment for coughs, gonorrhea, asthma, and indigestion, as a laxative, and to induce vomiting and increase urine flow.

BUTTERFLY MILKWEED   45

Asclepias tuberosa L.

OTHER COMMON NAMES: butterfly weed, Canada root, chigger flower, flux- root, Indian nosy, orange apocynum, orange milkweed, orangeroot, orange swallow-wort, pleurisy root, rubber root, ruber root, silkweed, swallow-wort, tu- berous-rooted swallow-wort, tuber root, white root, wind root, wind weed, wine tree.

PLANT DESCRIPTION: A slightly fuzzy, leafy perennial that grows to 3 feet in height. The leaves are 2 to 6 inches long, narrow, alternate, and have short stems. Bright orange flowers appear in a cluster. The seeds have white, silky hairs.

WHERE IT GROWS: Along the edges of forests, in sandy dry soils, pastures and roadsides, and gardens. New England, Michigan, Wisconsin, Minnesota, Nebras- ka, and Colorado; south to Florida and west to Texas and Arizona.

WHAT IS HARVESTED AND WHEN:
Roots, in the fall; leaves, as needed.

USES: A tea made of fresh leaves has been used in Appalachia to induce vomiting. Indians ate the raw root to treat bronchial ailments. The ground roots were used fresh or dry as a poultice for open sores. Taken internally, the root has been used to treat colic, hysteria, hemorrhage, gas, and weakness.

ANTELOPE HORN   46

Asclepiodora viridis (Walt.) Gray

OTHER COMMON NAMES:
spider milkweed

PLANT DESCRIPTION: A perennial with milky sap, growing to 2½ feet in height, resembling milkweed. The flowers are green and purple, 1 to 1½ inches across.

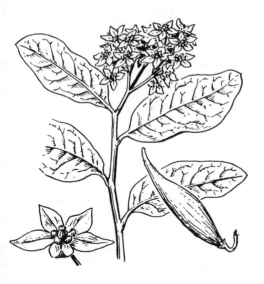

WHERE IT GROWS: At higher elevations in dry woods, fields, and prairies. New Mexico to Florida; north to South Carolina; west to Ohio and Missouri.

WHAT IS HARVESTED AND WHEN:
Roots, in the fall.

USES: Healing Herbs of the Upper Rio Grande, by L. S. M. Curtin, describes the many uses New Mexicans have for this plant. To relieve fever, they drink a decoction of the root in cold water. To relieve palpitation, the powdered root is rubbed over the heart area. A poultice of the powdered root is used to treat neck and rib pains and a tea made from it is used to alleviate asthma and shortness of breath.

COMMON PAWPAW   47

Asimina triloba (L.) Dunal.

OTHER COMMON NAMES: banana, custard apple, false banana, fetid shrub, jasmine, jasminier, North American pawpaw, papaw, wild banana.

PLANT DESCRIPTION: A tree growing to 40 feet in height. The leaves are oblong, 6 to 12 inches long. The flowers, on short stalks, are 2 inches across, dark

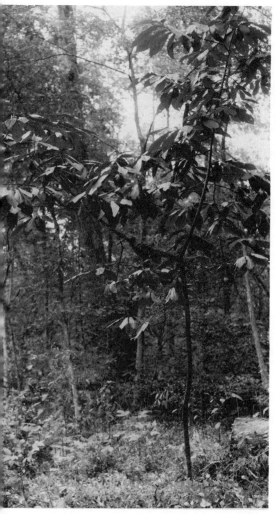

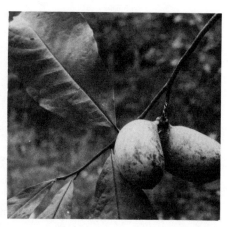

purple. The fruits are 3 to 7 inches long and 1 to 2 inches wide, yellow changing to dark brown, with flattened seeds.

WHERE IT GROWS: Deep, rich moist soils, rich bottomlands, and alluvial soils. New Jersey, New York, Illinois, Michigan, and Iowa south to Texas and Florida.

WHAT IS HARVESTED AND WHEN: Seeds, in fall or winter; fruit, when ripe, after a frost.

USES: The powdered seeds have been used to destroy head lice, the fruit juice to treat intestinal worms, and the seeds to induce vomiting.

PLAINS WILD INDIGO   48

Baptisia leucophaea Nutt..

OTHER COMMON NAME: cream-colored indigo.

PLANT DESCRIPTION: A hairy perennial growing to 2½ feet in height. The leaflets are up to 3 inches long; the flowers yellow to white, 1 to 1½ inches long.

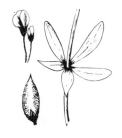

WHERE IT GROWS: Open, dry places. Oklahoma, Kansas, Texas, and Louisiana north to Michigan, Wisconsin, and Minnesota; rarely farther east.

WHAT IS HARVESTED AND WHEN: Leaves, when mature; roots, in the fall, from plants older than one year.

USES: A decoction of the leaves has been used as a stimulant and as an application for cuts and wounds. An infusion made from the root has been used as a remedy for typhoid and scarlet fever.

WILD INDIGO   49

Baptisia tinctoria (L.) R. Br.

OTHER COMMON NAMES: clover bloom, dyer's baptisia, false indigo, horsefly weed, indigo broom, indigo weed, rattlebush, rattleweed, yellow broom, yellow wild indigo.

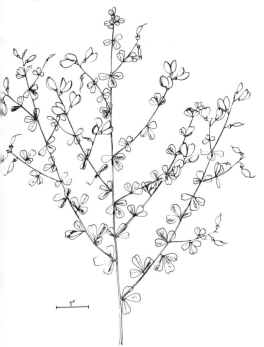

PLANT DESCRIPTION: A perennial that grows to 4 feet in height. The stem is erect and each branch has several whorls of clover-like leaflets. The yellow flowers, borne at the tops of highest branches, are ½ inch long, forming ½-inch brown pods.

WHERE IT GROWS: Dry woods and clearings. New York and Rhode Island, West Virginia south to Florida, and west to Indiana and Minnesota.

WHAT IS HARVESTED AND WHEN: Roots, in the fall.

USES: A century ago, people used to boil the root in water and take the liquid internally as a remedy for fever, scarlet fever, typhus, and sore throat. A poultice made from the root was used to treat ulcers. After the roots were steeped in water, open wounds were bathed in the liquid. The root has been considered laxative, astringent, and antiseptic, as well as useful in inducing vomiting.

Berberis vulgaris L.

OTHER COMMON NAMES: American barberry, barberry, common barberry, dragon grape, guild tree, jaundice barberry, jaundice berry, pepperidge bush, sow berry, wood sour, yellow root.

PLANT DESCRIPTION: A perennial shrub that grows to 8 feet in height. The leaves are small, green above, gray below; the leaves on young sprouts are very spiny. The flowers are yellow, the fruit scarlet to purple. The inner wood is yellow. Sharp spines occur at the nodes.

WHERE IT GROWS: Thickets and fence rows. New England, Delaware, and Pennsylvania, west to Minnesota, Iowa, and Missouri.

WHAT IS HARVESTED AND WHEN: Stem bark, root bark, and fruit, in the fall.

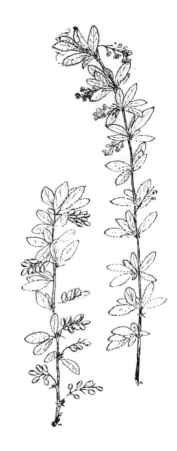

USES: The berries have been used to make a drink to reduce fever. A drink made from the root bark, steeped in beer, has been used to treat jaundice and hemorrhage. The fruit, which is rich in vitamin C, has been made into a confection and eaten to reduce fever and ease stomach distress. The bark has been used to treat dysentery and indigestion.

BLACK BIRCH 51

Betula lenta L.

OTHER COMMON NAMES: birch, cherry birch, mahogany birch, mountain mahogany, river birch, spice birch, sweet birch.

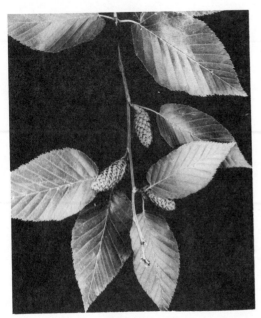

PLANT DESCRIPTION: A tree that grows to 75 feet in height, with dark, reddish brown bark, forming plates. Leaves 2½ to 5 inches long, with long hairs on the underside of the veins. The seeds are borne in catkins.

WHERE IT GROWS: Rich woods and uplands. New England south to Maryland, Tennessee, and Georgia.

WHAT IS HARVESTED AND WHEN: Leaves, twigs, and bark, as needed and available.

USES: A medicinal oil similar to oil of wintergreen has been extracted from the bark and small twigs and used to kill skin parasites. The dried leaves and twigs have been made into a dusting powder to soothe chafed skin. An infusion of the bark and twigs has been used to stimulate urine flow, to purify blood, and to treat rheumatism and gout.

PAPER BIRCH 52

Betula papyrifera Marsh.

OTHER COMMON NAMES: canoe birch, silver birch, white birch.

PLANT DESCRIPTION: A tree growing to 100 feet in height, with white, papery bark that peels into strips. The leaves are oval, 1½ to 4 inches long, and fuzzy on the underside.

WHERE IT GROWS: In woods and on the borders of lakes, streams, and swamps, often dispersed among other trees. Northeastern states, south to West Virginia, and west to Illinois, South Dakota, California, Oregon, and Washington.

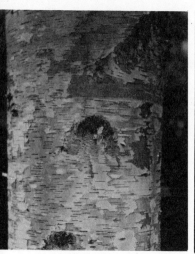
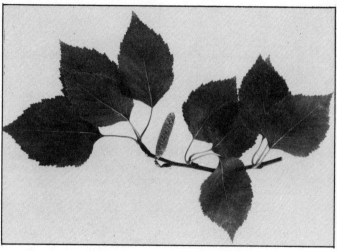

WHAT IS HARVESTED AND WHEN:
Leaves, when mature; roots and bark, as needed.

USES: Indians made a tea from the leaves, and a poultice of the boiled bark to treat bruises, wounds, and burns. The ashes were used to remove scabs from cuts and wounds. The root was often used in unpalatable foods to disguise the taste. Some Indians took the new soft wood, chopped it very fine, and mixed it with tobacco. Occasionally the sap has been collected and made into vinegar.

BEES RAPE   53

Brassica rapa L.

OTHER COMMON NAMES: Bergeman's cabbage, field mustard, rape, rutabaga, summer rape, wild navette, wild turnip.

PLANT DESCRIPTION: A slender, erect annual growing to 3 feet in height. The leaves are 3 to 6 inches long, lobed. The yellow flowers are about 1/3 inch across.

WHERE IT GROWS: Fields and gardens, roadsides. Throughout the United States.

WHAT IS HARVESTED AND WHEN:
Seeds, in summer.

USES: The use of a "mustard plaster," made of a flour from the seeds of this plant, plus water, wrapped in a brown bag, and applied to the chest for colds, fever, and flu, is familiar to many of us who grew up in the twenties. The seeds have been used to induce vomiting, as an aid to digestion, and as a laxative.

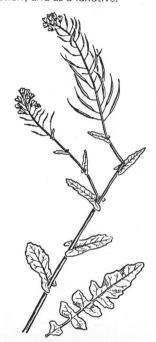

MARIJUANA   54

Cannabis sativa L.

OTHER COMMON NAMES: cannabis, cherry, common hemp, gunjok, hashish, hemp, hempweed, Indian hemp, loco weed, maryjane, pot, neckweed.

PLANT DESCRIPTION: An annual growing to 16 feet in height. The male and female plants are usually separate. The leaves are alternate, narrow, long-stemmed, and large-toothed, with several leaflets.

WHERE IT GROWS: Old fields, cultivated fields, vacant city lots, and stream banks. Almost all parts of the United States.

WHAT IS HARVESTED AND WHEN: Flowering top of the female plant, in late summer; leaves, as they mature.

USES: Once used as a source of fiber for hemp, this common introduced plant is taken as a drug in several ways (smoking, etc.) to create a feeling of euphoria, well-being, and relaxation. The growth, possession, and use of the plant are illegal in many countries. In India, thugs would give their victims one form of the plant (hashish) so as to drug them before robbing them. The plant has been used medically to treat nervous disorders, tetanus, gonorrhea, depression, and blad-

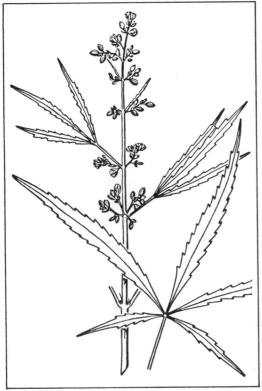

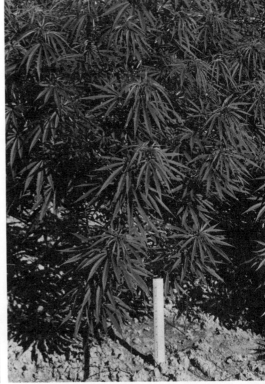

der inflammation. One old family medical guide recommended it for discouraging masturbation. In Kentucky, a friend told us that when he was a youngster his neighbors who were too poor to buy bourbon would smoke a "reefer" of marijuana instead.

SHEPHERD'S PURSE   55

Capsella bursa-pastoris (L.) Medic.

OTHER COMMON NAMES: caseweed, shepherd's-bag, shovelweed.

PLANT DESCRIPTION: An annual growing to 20 inches in height, originating from a basal rosette of leaves. The small, white flowers at the end of the stems mature into the flat, triangular, heart-shaped pods about ¼ inch long from which the plant gets its name.

WHERE IT GROWS: Generally in open sunny areas, pastures, old fields, and empty lots. Throughout the United States.

WHAT IS HARVESTED AND WHEN: Plants and their juices, as needed.

USES: The juice of the plant on a ball of cotton was used to plug into nostrils to stop nosebleed. People also used it to clear phlegm from the chest, to increase urine flow and menstrual flow, and to correct a vitamin C shortage. As a decoction, it has been used to treat hemorrhoids, diarrhea, and bloody urine:

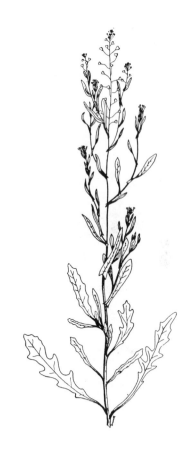

SAFFLOWER   56

Carthamus tinctorius L.

OTHER COMMON NAMES: American saffron, azafran, bastard saffron, false saffron, saffron.

PLANT DESCRIPTION: An annual with alternate spiny leaves, up to 3 feet in height. The flowers are orange-yellow; the seeds, white and shiny.

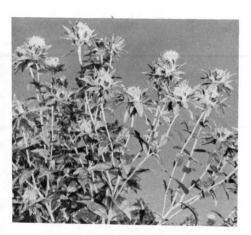

WHERE IT GROWS: Wild in Afghanistan; in the U.S. under cultivation, mainly in California.

WHAT IS HARVESTED AND WHEN: Flowers, at maturity; seeds, when available; entire plant, when in bloom.

USES: Indians drank a tea made with the flowers to counteract skin eruptions caused by contact with poisonous plants. A paste made of the flowers and water was applied to boils. The petals were boiled with lamb and eaten to strengthen the heart. Safflower was used as a laxative, to induce perspiration, and to stimulate menstrual flow. Among New Mexicans the plant is used to dry up the skin symptoms of measles. They also soak the flowers in water until the water is visibly yellow, then drink the decoction to reduce fever.

WILD SENNA   57

Cassia marilandica L.

OTHER COMMON NAMES: American senna, cassia, locust plant, Maryland cassia.

PLANT DESCRIPTION: A perennial growing to 4 feet in height. The leaves are light green; the leaflets in five to ten pairs, 1 to 2 inches long. The flowers are bright yellow; the pod long and narrow, flat, 4 inches long.

WHERE IT GROWS: Dry roadsides and thickets. Pennsylvania to Kansas and Iowa, south to Texas and Florida.

WHAT IS HARVESTED AND WHEN: Leaves, when mature; roots, in the fall.

USES: Indians used the bruised roots as a poultice for sores, a decoction of the roots for treating fever, and the leaves as a mild laxative. The pioneers took senna as a laxative, and it is widely used for the same purpose today.

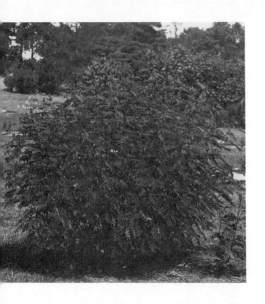
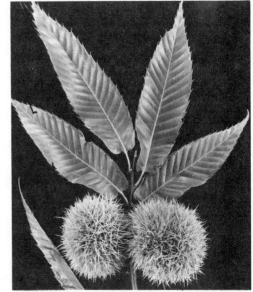
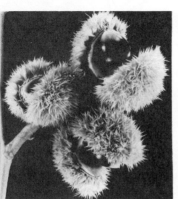
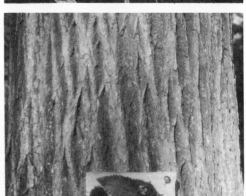

AMERICAN CHESTNUT 58

Castanea dentata (Marsh.) Borkh.

OTHER COMMON NAMES: chestnut, prickly bur, sweet chestnut.

PLANT DESCRIPTION: A tree growing to 100 feet in height, with leaves 5 to 10 inches long, margins deeply serrated, forward-pointed. Two to three nuts are found together, ½ inch to 1 inch in diameter, brown, flattened on one side.

WHERE IT GROWS: Rich woods at various elevations, in rather acid soils.

The species has been almost destroyed by a fungus disease, and only shoots from old stumps survive. At one time the tree was abundant in the area from Maine to Michigan, south to Delaware, Illinois, Kentucky, and the Appalachian area, Alabama, Georgia, Florida, Mississippi, Arkansas, and Texas.

WHAT IS HARVESTED AND WHEN: Leaves. at any time during the growing season; bark, at any time.

USES: Indians made a tea from the leaves to treat whooping cough; and the same tea has been used as a sedative and tonic. The bark was used to treat worms and dysentery.

COMMON CATALPA   59

Catalpa bignonioides Walt.

OTHER COMMON NAMES: beantree; candle-tree, catawba, catawba-tree, cigar-tree, Indian-bean, Indian cigar-tree, smoking bean.

PLANT DESCRIPTION: A tree growing to 60 feet in height. The leaves are 6 to 8 inches long, sometimes with 2 lobes, fuzzy beneath, and have a disagreeable odor when crushed. The flowers are in long clusters, each flower 2 inches across, white with yellow and purple-brown markings. The pods are dark brown, thin, up to 15 inches long.

WHERE IT GROWS: Barnyard areas, wood lots, roadsides, gardens, and stream banks. Eastern United States from New England south to Kentucky, Tennessee, Georgia, Alabama, Louisiana, and Mississippi.

59

60

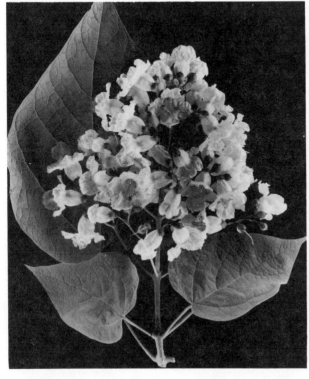

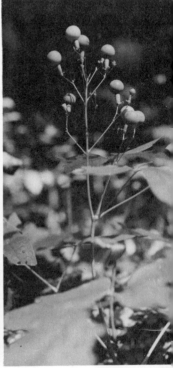

WHAT IS HARVESTED AND WHEN:
Pods, in late summer and fall; bark and leaves, as needed.

USES: The bark has been used to expel intestinal worms; the leaves have been applied as a poultice to skin wounds and abrasions. The seeds have been used to induce vomiting and to treat intestinal worms. The bark, in decoction, is a mild laxative.

BLUE COHOSH   60

Caulophyllum thalictroides (L.) Michx.

OTHER COMMON NAMES: blueberry, blueberry cohosh, blueberry root, blue ginseng, papoose root, squaw root, yellow ginseng.

PLANT DESCRIPTION: A perennial that grows to 3 feet in height. The leaflets are either two- or three-lobed. In spring, the plant sends up a stem of yellowish green flowers.

WHERE IT GROWS: Hardwood forests and mountain glades. New England to the mountains of Appalachia and south to South Carolina.

WHAT IS HARVESTED AND WHEN:
Roots, in the fall.

USES: The powdered root was taken by Indian women to induce menstrual flow and to hasten childbirth. A root tea was used to strengthen the stomach and to treat venereal disease. The root was also used to increase perspiration, relieve spasms, and treat sore throat, colic, and rheumatism.

NEW JERSEY TEA   61

Ceanothus americanus L.

OTHER COMMON NAMES: Jersey tea ceanothus, New Jersey tea tree, red root, wild snowball.

PLANT DESCRIPTION: A shrub that grows to 3 feet in height. The leaves are finely toothed, dark green above, pale green below. White flowers on long stalks appear in the upper part of the plant. The root is dark red.

WHERE IT GROWS: Dry areas, open woods, rocky ledges, and hardwood forests. Maine to Minnesota, south to Florida, Alabama, and Texas.

WHAT IS HARVESTED AND WHEN:
Roots, in the fall; leaves, when they have reached full growth; seeds, in the fall.

USES: During the American Revolution,

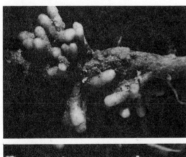

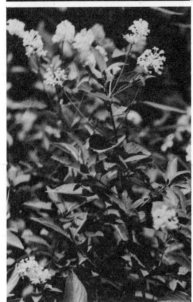

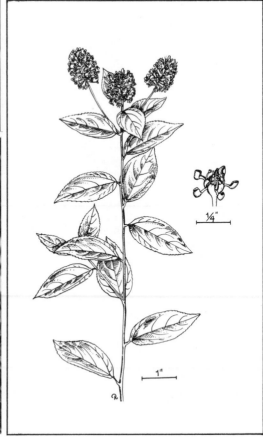

the leaves were used as a substitute for tea. A decoction of leaves and seeds has been used to cure ulcerated sore throat. Indians used a decoction of the roots as a wash for cancer and syphilis. The plant has been used to treat gonorrhea, dysentery, and eye disease in children. The root is reported to be a stimulant, a sedative, and a means of loosening phlegm.

BITTERSWEET   62

Celastrus scandens L.

OTHER COMMON NAMES: climbing bittersweet, climbing orange-root, false bittersweet, fever twig, fever-twitch, wax-work.

PLANT DESCRIPTION: A twining plant growing to over 25 feet in length. The leaves are 2 to 5 inches long, 1 inch wide. The flowers are greenish and very small. The seed capsules are globe-shaped, orange to yellow, and about 1/3 inch in diameter.

WHERE IT GROWS: Dense, moist thickets, fence rows, waste grounds, road-sides. New England through the Appalachian Mountains, south to Georgia, Alabama, and Louisiana, and west to Oklahoma.

WHAT IS HARVESTED AND WHEN: Root bark, in the fall.

USES: The bark of the root has been taken internally to induce vomiting, to quiet disturbed people, to treat venereal diseases, and to increase urine flow. As an ointment mixed with grease it has been used to treat skin cancers, tumors, burns, and swellings. A decoction of the root bark has been used to induce menstrual flow and perspiration. The attractive orange fruits are a common sight at roadside stands in the Appalachian region and are used for dry flower arrangements.

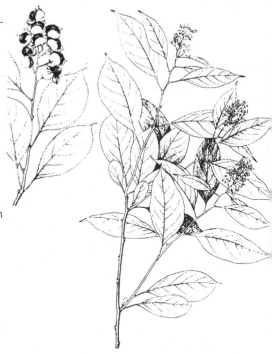

COMMON BUTTONBUSH   63

Cephalanthus occidentalis L.

OTHER COMMON NAMES: buttonbush, button-willow, crane-willow, crooked wood, globe flower, honey-balls, mountain globe-flower, pin-ball, pond dogwood, river-bush, swamp dog wood, swamp wood.

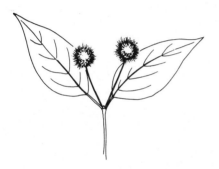

PLANT DESCRIPTION: A deciduous shrub ranging from 5 to 20 feet in height. The leaves are 3 to 6 inches long, opposite, and shiny above. The flowers are yellowish to white 1/3 to 1/2 inch long, and occur in dense heads.

WHERE IT GROWS: Swamps and low ground near lakes and ponds. Michigan, Minnesota, Nebraska, Kansas, Oklahoma, Texas, New Mexico, Arizona, and California, and from New York south to Florida.

WHAT IS HARVESTED AND WHEN: Bark, at any season; inner bark, in spring or fall; roots, at any time.

USES: Indians induced vomiting with a tea made from the inner bark. The bark was used as a laxative and tonic, also in the form of a tea, and has been chewed to relieve toothache. A tincture of the bark has been used to treat fever, coughs, and venereal disease. The root, boiled and mixed with honey to make a syrup, has been used to treat pleurisy.

FAIRYWAND   64

Chamaelirium luteum (L.) Gray

OTHER COMMON NAMES: blazing star, devil's bit, false unicorn, false unicorn root, grub root, helonias, rattlesnake root, star root, starwort.

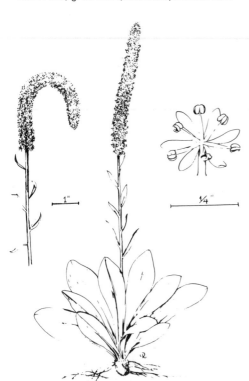

PLANT DESCRIPTION: A perennial that grows to a height of 4 feet and originates from a rosette of basal leaves. Male and female plants are separate. Male flowers are white, female flowers green.

WHERE IT GROWS: Damp pine barrens, upland forests, bogs, and wet places in meadows and woodlands. New England, New York, Ohio, Michigan, and Illinois, south to Florida and Arkansas.

WHAT IS HARVESTED AND WHEN: Rootstock, in the fall.

USES: The powdered roots were used in pioneer times to treat uterine disorders, pain in the head, pain in the side and loins, poor appetite, depression, and colic. The rootstock was used to treat intestinal worms, to remedy vitamin C deficiency, and to induce increased urine flow, vomiting, and saliva flow. Indians chewed the root to relieve coughs and check miscarriage.

Chelone glabra L.

OTHER COMMON NAMES: balmony, bitter herb, fishmouth, salt-rheum weed, shellflower, smooth snakehead, snakehead, snakemouth, true snakehead, turtle bloom, turtlehead.

PLANT DESCRIPTION: A perennial that grows to 3 feet in height, with narrow, opposite leaves and rose-white flowers 1 inch long. It produces a many-seeded capsule.

WHERE IT GROWS: Low grounds, swampy areas, stream borders, wet forested areas, and woodlands, New England west to Minnesota and south to Georgia, Alabama, and Mississippi.

WHAT IS HARVESTED AND WHEN: Leaves, in the spring; flowering aboveground parts, in late summer to early fall.

USES: The powdered leaves, as well as the entire plant, have been used as a laxative and tonic, and to treat worms and jaundice.

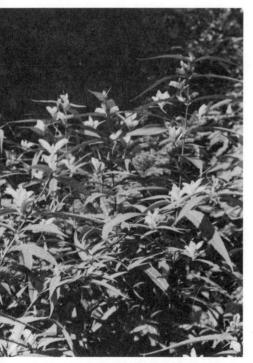

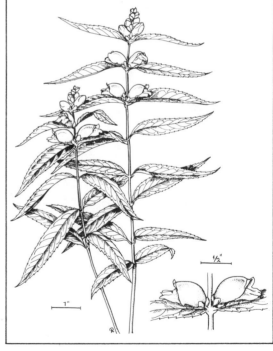

LAMB'S QUARTERS   66

Chenopodium album L.

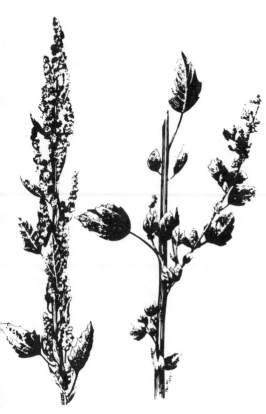

OTHER COMMON NAMES: bacon-weed, fat hen, goosefoot, muchweed, pigweed, smooth pigweed, white cheno-podium, white goosefoot, wild spinach, wormseed.

PLANT DESCRIPTION: An annual growing to 4 feet in height, with a whitish, fuzzy surface. The lower leaf surface is whiter than the upper. The flowers are greenish, arising in spikes from the upper leaf axils.

WHERE IT GROWS: Gardens, fields, waste grounds, dry woods, and old fields. All parts of the United States.

WHAT IS HARVESTED AND WHEN: Entire plant, at full bloom; leaves, when mature, or very young leaves in the spring; seeds, in summer.

USES: The young leaves make an excel-lent vegetable dish, high in vitamin C and mildly laxative. In times of famine in Europe, the seeds were mixed with wheat to make the wheat crop go further. In-dians made a tea of the leaves and plant to relieve stomach pains.

MEXICAN TEA   67

Chenopodium ambrosioides L.

OTHER COMMON NAMES: ambrosia, ambrosia-like chenopodium, American wormseed, Jerusalem oak, Jerusalem oak seed, Jerusalem tea, jesuit tea, Spanish tea, stickweed, stinking weed, wild worm-seed, wormseed, wormseed goosefoot.

PLANT DESCRIPTION: An annual that grows to 4 feet in height. The branches sprout in numbers from the base; the leaves are alternate and up to 5 inches long. Small, greenish flowers appear in the axils of the leaves.

WHERE IT GROWS: Old fields, waste places, and cultivated areas. Almost all states.

WHAT IS HARVESTED AND WHEN: Fruit, in summer; entire plant, in the fall.

USES: In New Mexico, this plant has been used as a tea to hasten milk flow from nursing mothers and to relieve post-delivery pains. In Mexico, it is cooked and eaten to treat intestinal worms. The fruit is the source of chenopodium oil, used to treat intestinal worms in humans and animals. Considered a slightly narcotic plant, it has been used both to induce menstrual flow and to reduce profuse and painful menstrual flow, as well as to treat nervous conditions.

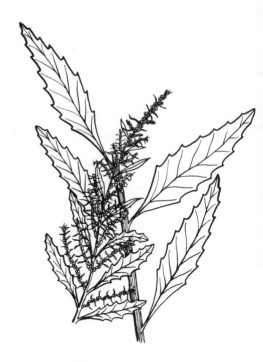

SPOTTED WINTERGREEN 68

Chimaphila maculata (L.) Pursh.

OTHER COMMON NAMES: dragon's tongue, pepsissewa, ratsbane, rheumatism root, spotted pipsissewa, wild arsenic, wintergreen.

PLANT DESCRIPTION: An evergreen perennial that grows to 12 inches in height. The leaves are dark, shiny green, wedge-shaped. The flowers are ½ inch in size, flesh-colored, with small spots of violet color within.

WHERE IT GROWS: Forests and dry woods. New Hampshire to Michigan and Illinois; south to Georgia, Alabama, and the Appalachian highlands of Tennessee, Kentucky, and West Virginia; west to California.

WHAT IS HARVESTED AND WHEN: Leaves and fruit, as needed.

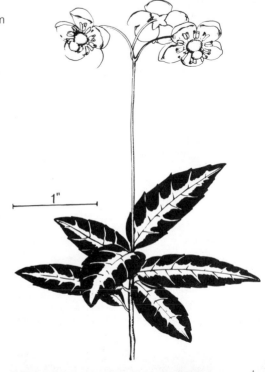

1"

USES: The leaves and fruit have been used to increase urine flow, as a tonic, and for treating diarrhea, rheumatism, syphilis, skin eruptions, nervous disorders, and ulcers.

COMMON PIPSISSEWA   69

Chimaphila umbellata Bart. L.

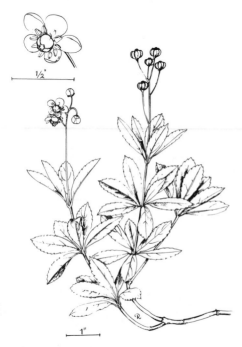

OTHER COMMON NAMES: bitter wintergreen, fragrant wintergreen, ground holly, king's cure, love-in-winter, noble pine, pine tulip, pipsissewa, prince's pine, princess pine, pyrole, rheumatism weed, waxflower, wintergreen.

PLANT DESCRIPTION: A small evergreen perennial that grows to 10 inches in height. The leaves are dark green, blunt-toothed, and wedge-shaped. The flowers are about ½ inch in size, flesh-colored with violet pollen sacs.

WHERE IT GROWS: A shade-loving plant found in coniferous and hardwood forests and acid woodlands, in dry woods, and often in sandy soil. New England to Minnesota, Ohio, and Michigan; south to Virginia, West Virginia, and North Carolina; west to Oregon, Washington, California, and Colorado.

WHAT IS HARVESTED AND WHEN: Leaves, preferably during the growing season; fruits, from late summer as long as they remain on the plant; entire plant, when in flower.

USES: This plant was widely used by Indians. They made hot infusions of it to induce perspiration in the treatment of typhus. The berries were eaten for stomach disorders, and a tea of the leaves was used for the same purpose. During the Civil War, a decoction of the plant was used as a tonic and to increase urine flow, and as a tea, to treat rheumatism and kidney problems.

Chionanthus virginicus L.

OTHER COMMON NAMES: American fringe, American fringe tree, flowering ash, graybeard, graybeard tree, old man's beard, poison ash, shavings, snowdrop tree, snowflowers, snowflower tree, white ash, white fringe, white fringe tree.

PLANT DESCRIPTION: A tree that grows to 35 feet in height and produces many white flowers on long stems, in groups. The berries are purple, fleshy, and round.

WHERE IT GROWS: In rich, moist soils, on banks of streams in damp woods and thickets, bluffs and woods. Southern Pennsylvania to northeastern Kentucky, south to the southern Appalachians, Florida, and the Gulf states, to Arkansas, Oklahoma, and Texas.

WHAT IS HARVESTED AND WHEN: Root bark and trunk bark, in spring or fall; flowers, in late summer.

USES: In Appalachia, a decoction of boiled bark is used to treat skin inflammations. Indians boiled the bark in water and used the liquid to bathe wounds, also to treat fever associated with malaria. Pioneers applied a poultice of crushed bark to cuts and bruises. The leaves and flowers have been used to treat inflammations and sores, ulcers in the mouth and throat, and diarrhea.

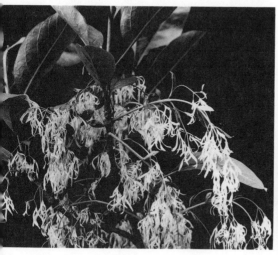
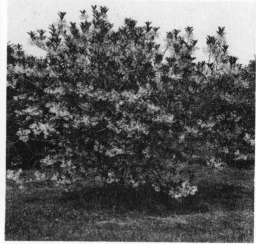

Chrysanthemum parthenium (L.) Bernh.

OTHER COMMON NAME: chrysanthemum.

PLANT DESCRIPTION: A much-branched perennial, up to 3 feet in height, sometimes with yellow foliage. The flowers are white and yellow, and occur in tight clusters.

WHERE IT GROWS: Dry areas, waste places, roadsides, and borders of woods. Throughout the United States.

WHAT IS HARVESTED AND WHEN: Leaves and flowers, as available.

USES: Children with colic have been given the leaves to chew. A tea made of the dry, ground leaves is used to treat bad colds, indigestion, and diarrhea. To relieve constipation, a suppository made of dry leaves, honey, and soap has been used in New Mexico. The dried flowers are used to treat indigestion, kill intestinal worms, induce menstrual flow, and bring about abortion.

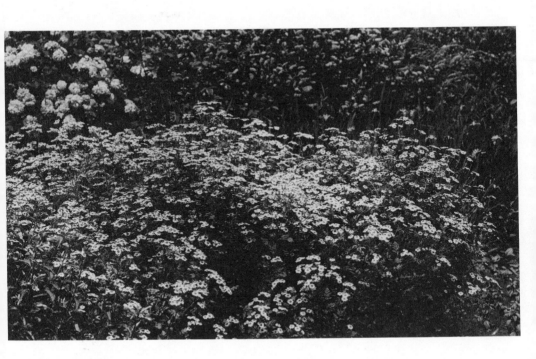

AMERICAN BUGBANE   72

Cimicifuga americana Michx.

OTHER COMMON NAMES: bugbane, mountain bugbane, mountain rittletop, summer cohosh.

PLANT DESCRIPTION: A perennial plant that grows to 4 feet in height. Small white flowers are borne on short lateral spikes, plus a terminal spike.

WHERE IT GROWS: Moist woods in mountain areas. New England, Pennsylvania, Wisconsin, south to Georgia, North Carolina, Tennessee, and Kentucky, and west to Missouri.

WHAT IS HARVESTED AND WHEN: Roots, in early fall when plant has bloomed.

USES: A weak decoction of the root was used in the 1800's to treat skin rash. The dried powdered root has been used to repel vermin and to treat rattlesnake bites. The root was believed to be effective in relieving the pains of childbirth, and in the treatment of rheumatism, hysteria, and lung inflammations.

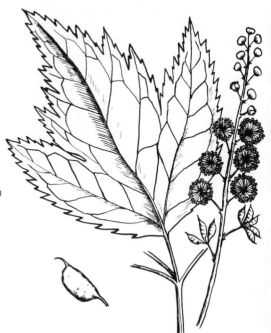

COHOSH BUGBANE   73

Cimicifuga racemosa (L.) Nutt.

OTHER COMMON NAMES: battle weed, black cohosh, black snakeroot, blueberry, blue ginseng, bugbane, cohosh, columbine leaved leontice, cordate rattle-top, false cohosh, heart-leaved rattle-top, heart-leaved snakeroot, meadow rue leontice, papoose root, rattle root, rattlesnake root, rattle-top, rattleweed, richweed, squaw root, yellow ginseng.

PLANT DESCRIPTION: A perennial shrub that grows to 9 feet or more in height. The leaf has two to five leaflets, and the plant is topped with a slender spike of small white or yellowish flowers. The rhizome is gnarled and twisted.

WHERE IT GROWS: Rich open woods. Massachusetts to New York, Ohio, Indi-

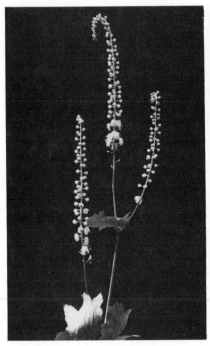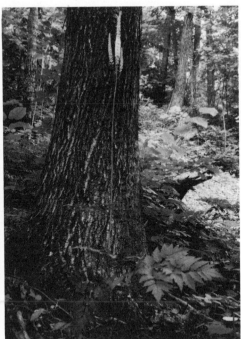

ana, and Missouri, south to South Carolina, Georgia, and Tennessee.

WHAT IS HARVESTED AND WHEN:
Rhizomes and roots, in the fall.

USES: In Appalachia, a tea made from the root is used as a treatment for sore throat. Indians used a decoction of the root for rheumatism, kidney trouble, and general malaise. They also used the rhizomes to treat women's ailments, to promote perspiration, and to treat malaria. The colonists used it for yellow fever, itching, bronchitis, nervous diseases, uterine disorders, and snakebite.

CAMPHORTREE   74

Cinnamomum camphora (L.) Nees and Eberm.

OTHER COMMON NAME: camphor laurel.

PLANT DESCRIPTION: A tree that grows to 40 feet in height, with an enlarged base. Both leaves and twigs have a strong camphor smell. The leaves are 2 to 5 inches long, smooth and shiny above, whitish beneath. The flowers are yellow, the fruit 3/8 inch in diameter.

WHERE IT GROWS: Dry, sunny sites. California and Florida.

WHAT IS HARVESTED AND WHEN:
Twigs and leaves, at any time during the growing season.

USES: This native of China is the source of camphor, which is somewhat antiseptic, acts as a circulatory stimulant, and has a calming effect in cases of hysteria, general nervousness, and neuralgia. The distilled oil has been used to treat diarrhea, rheumatism, and muscular pains. Small doses act to stimulate respiration; large doses can be toxic by stopping respiration. Doctors have disagreed as to whether camphor will stop heart fibrillation, and whether it is a heart stimulant, as is widely believed in Europe.

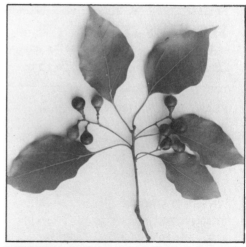

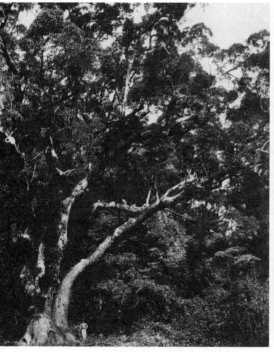

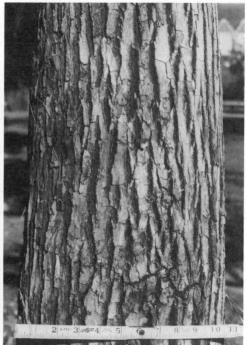

Cirsium flodmani (Rydb.) Arthur

PLANT DESCRIPTION: A biennial plant arising from a basal rosette to a height of 2½ feet. The leaves are whitish below, gray and fuzzy above. The flowers are purple.

WHERE IT GROWS: Fields, pastures, meadows, and moist areas. New York and New England to Iowa, Nebraska, Colorado, and Utah.

WHAT IS HARVESTED AND WHEN: Roots, leaves, flowers, and stems, as needed.

USES: The juice of the leaves and stems has been used as a scalp tonic to restore falling hair. The plant has been boiled in milk and the liquid drunk to treat dysentery. The juice of the roots has been used by New Mexicans to relieve earache. They also use a decoction of the flowers to treat gonorrhea.

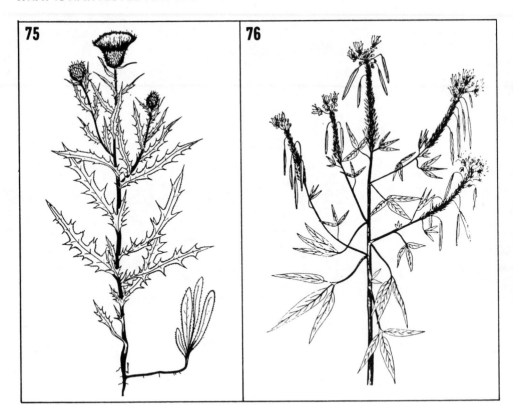

STINKING CLOVER　　76

Cleome serrulata Pursh.

OTHER COMMON NAMES: bee spider flower, guaco, Rocky Mountain bee plant.

PLANT DESCRIPTION: An annual growing to 3 feet in height. The leaflets are ¾ to 1½ inches long; the flowers are usually purplish rose.

WHERE IT GROWS: Prairies and damp, waste places. Missouri, Kansas, Illinois, Ohio; Arizona and New Mexico to Oregon and Washington.

WHAT IS HARVESTED AND WHEN: Leaves, when mature; flowers, as they appear.

USES: A poultice made of the crushed leaves has been used to reduce swellings. The flowers have been boiled with rusty iron and the liquid drunk as a treatment for anemia.

BLESSED THISTLE　　77

Cnicus benedictus L.

OTHER COMMON NAMES: bitter thistle, bitterweed, blessed carduus, carduus, cursed thistle, holy thistle, our-lady's thistle, St. Benedict's thistle, spotted carduus, spotted thistle.

PLANT DESCRIPTION: This annual grows to 2 feet in height and has spiny, toothed, lobed leaves. The plant produces many-flowered yellow heads.

WHERE IT GROWS: Roadsides and waste places. Eastern United States and parts of the Southwest.

WHAT IS HARVESTED AND WHEN: Leaves and flowering tops, when in full bloom; seeds, at maturity.

USES: The seeds have been used to induce vomiting. Indians used an infusion of the tops as a contraceptive measure. In

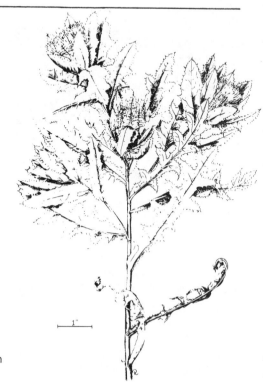

the last century, people used such an infusion to treat internal cancer, to increase sweating and urine flow, to expel worms, and to treat fever, hysteria, liver ailments, and inflammations of the respiratory system.

SEAGRAPE 78

Coccoloba uvifera (L.) Jacq.

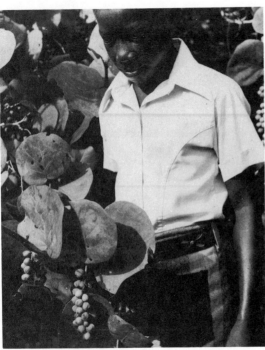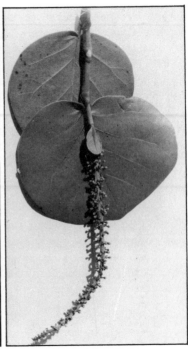

OTHER COMMON NAMES: grape-tree, platter-leaf, seaside plum, uva de playa.

PLANT DESCRIPTION: An evergreen shrub or tree growing to 20 feet in height. The leaves are almost round, 1½ to 8 inchee across, heart-shaped at the base, leathery and glossy. The flowers are white, borne in dense clusters. The fruits are dark purple, thin-fleshed, and clustered like grapes.

WHERE IT GROWS: Along shore lines and at the edge of bodies of salt water. Florida, Puerto Rico, and the Virgin Islands.

WHAT IS HARVESTED AND WHEN: Bark, as needed; fruits, at summer's end; roots, in the spring or fall.

USES: The fruits, tasty but not filling, have been used to reduce fever. The roots have been used to treat diarrhea. The bark yields an extract known as "Jamaica kino," used to treat dysentery.

Collinsonia canadensis L.

OTHER COMMON NAMES: broadleaf collinsonia, Canadian collinsonia, citronella, heal-all, horse balm, horseweed, knob grass, knobroot, ox balm, richweed, stone root.

PLANT DESCRIPTION: A perennial that grows to 3 feet in height, with opposite, coarsely toothed, ovate leaves. The rhizomes are thick and woody, the flowers strongly scented and lemon yellow.

WHERE IT GROWS: Rich, moist woods. Massachusetts, Vermont, and New York west to Wisconsin and south to Florida and Arkansas.

WHAT IS HARVESTED AND WHEN: Entire plant, during flowering; roots, in the fall.

USES: A tincture of the root added to cider has been used to treat bodily water accumulation. People in Appalachia make a tea from the plant and use it to treat headaches, cramps, and indigestion.

A drop or two of the tincture in water, taken three times daily, was once used to treat hemorrhoids. The tincture has also been used to treat respiratory diseases.

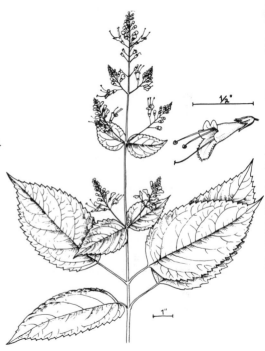

SWEET FERN 80

Comptonia peregrina (L.) Coult.

OTHER COMMON NAMES: Canadian sweetgale, fern bush, ferngale, ferngate, meadow fern, shrubby fern, shrubby-sweet fern, spleen fern, spleenwort fern, sweet bush, sweet ferry.

PLANT DESCRIPTION: A sweet-smelling perennial shrub that grows to 3 to 5 feet in height. The leaves are alternate, 3 to 6 inches long, linear, and deeply notched. The flower is a fuzzy catkin, followed by shiny brown nutlets ¼ inch long.

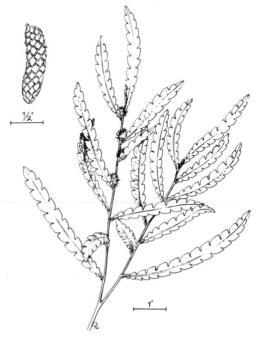

WHERE IT GROWS: Sunny areas such as pastures, dry open woods, and abandoned fields. New England south to Virginia, West Virginia, Ohio, Georgia to Tennessee, west to Indiana, Illinois, and Minnesota.

WHAT IS HARVESTED AND WHEN:
Leaves, plant, during the growing season.

USES: The leaves were boiled by Indians to make a poultice that was tied to the cheek to relieve toothache. A decoction of the plant was used to treat diarrhea, rheumatism, colic, and weakness following fever.

GOLDTHREAD 81

Coptis groenlandica (Oeder) Fernald

OTHER COMMON NAME: cankerroot.

PLANT DESCRIPTION: A perennial about 6 inches in height, with shiny, evergreen leaves. The white flowers are usually solitary.

WHERE IT GROWS: Wet places, bogs, woods, and swamps. New England, Tennessee, Kentucky, North Carolina, Ohio, and Indiana.

WHAT IS HARVESTED AND WHEN:
Roots, as needed, entire plant, when in bloom.

USES: The plant was used in New England to treat fever blisters in children's mouths, also to treat indigestion and restore strength after prolonged illness.

Indians chewed the roots to treat mouth sores and made a tea of the plant to use as a wash for eye irritations and mouth sores.

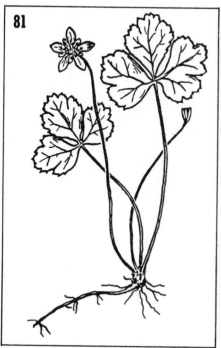

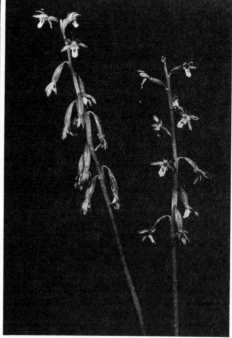

SPOTTED CHATELAIN   82

Corallorhiza maculata Raf.

OTHER COMMON NAMES: spotted coral-root, spotted coral-weed.

PLANT DESCRIPTION: A perennial about 1 foot in height, lacking green foliage. The flowers are yellow, or brown to purple, or white spotted with red or purple.

WHERE IT GROWS: Dry woods. New England to North Carolina, Tennessee,

Kentucky, Ohio, Indiana, Wisconsin, Minnesota, South Dakota, Colorado, and California.

WHAT IS HARVESTED AND WHEN: Roots and stalks, as needed.

USES: The dried stalks have been used to make a tea for strengthening patients suffering from pneumonia. The roots have been used as a sedative, to kill worms, and to increase perspiration.

FLOWERING DOGWOOD   83

Cornus florida L.

OTHER COMMON NAMES: arrow-wood, bitter red berry, boxwood, common dogwood, cornel, dog tree, dogwood, false box, false box dogwood, false boxwood, Florida dogwood, flowering cornel, great-flowered dogwood, New England boxwood, Virginia dogwood, white cornel.

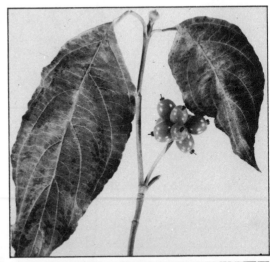

PLANT DESCRIPTION: A shrub or small tree that grows to 15 feet in height. The flowers are greenish yellow to creamy white, without stems. The fruit is bright red, sometimes yellow, borne in dense clusters.

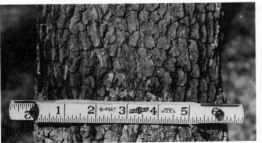

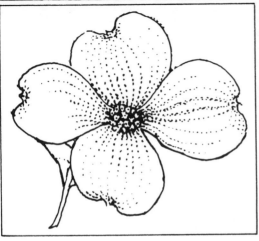

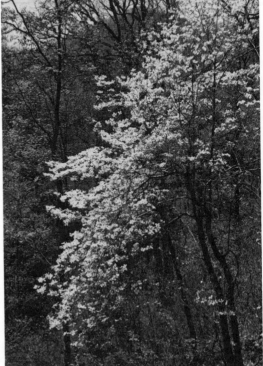

WHERE IT GROWS: Acid woods, rich shady areas, and moist forests. New England west to Michigan, Illinois, and Kansas, and south to Texas and Florida.

WHAT IS HARVESTED AND WHEN: Root bark, flowers, and inner bark, in early spring or late fall; fruit, in late fall and early winter.

USES: Indians boiled the bark in water and rubbed aching muscles with the liquid. In colonial times, the flowers, fruit, and bark were steeped in warm water and the bitter brew was used to treat fevers and malaria. The inner bark has been boiled to make a tea used for dysentery. In the 1800's the root bark was used in place of quinine to treat malaria. The bark has been used for treating worms, cholera, sore mouth, jaundice and liver ailments.

CYPRESS 84

Cupressus arizonica Greene

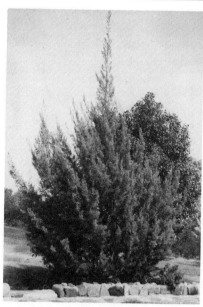 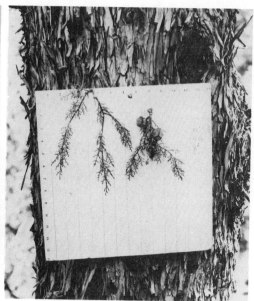

OTHER COMMON NAMES: Arizona cypress, smooth Arizona cypress, smooth cypress.

PLANT DESCRIPTION: An evergreen tree growing to 60 feet in height. The outer bark is thin, dark brownish, with vertical fissures. The seeds are winged.

WHERE IT GROWS: Mountainsides at elevations of 4,500 to 6,500 feet. Southern Arizona and New Mexico.

WHAT IS HARVESTED AND WHEN:
Fruit, in the fall; leaves and stems, as needed.

USES: The vapor of the burning leaves was once used as an aid in childbirth, to help in removing the afterbirth; shrink the womb, and increase urine flow. The pounded leaves were applied as a poultice to treat ringworm, tumors, and ulcers, as well as toothache and skin inflammations. The baked stems were applied to burns and damaged skin areas. The fruit has been used to ease stomach gas.

DODDER   85

Cuscuta megalocarpa Rydb.

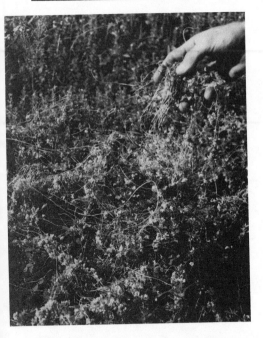

OTHER COMMON NAMES: golden thread, love-vine, strangle weed, yerba mate, yerba sin raiz.

PLANT DESCRIPTION: A parasitic annual with slender, twining stems that may be yellow, white, or red. The leaves are hardly visible, the whitish flowers 1/8 inch long in dense clusters.

WHERE IT GROWS: Climbing over other plants, wild and cultivated, usually in open areas or in partial shade. Colorado, Wyoming, New Mexico, and Minnesota to the eastern states.

WHAT IS HARVESTED AND WHEN:
Entire plant, when in flower.

USES: Indians used the plants in a bath for treatment of tuberculosis. Early settlers put their fevered children in the same kind of bath. A poultice of the plant has been used to treat insect stings. Indians believed the plant to be a useful contraceptive and gave it to their women. It has also been considered a bile stimulant and a laxative.

YELLOW LADY'S SLIPPER   86

Cypripedium calceolus L.

OTHER COMMON NAMES: American valerian, lady-slipper, nerve root, small-golden slipper, small moccasin flower, small yellow lady's slipper, yellow Indian shoe, yellow moccasin.

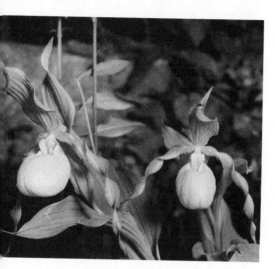

PLANT DESCRIPTION: A highly aromatic perennial from 6 to 24 inches in height. The leaves are ovate and alternate, originating around the stem. The saclike flowers range in color from greenish yellow to purplish brown.

WHERE IT GROWS: Bogs, moist woods, and shady areas. New England to South Carolina, and Louisiana, and west to New Mexico.

WHAT IS HARVESTED AND WHEN: Roots and rhizomes, in fall or spring.

USES: In Appalachia, a root tea is used as a remedy for headaches and jangling nerves. A teaspoonful of the powdered root in sugar water has been used as a sedative, to promote sleep, and to allay pain.

Datura meteloides DC.

OTHER COMMON NAMES: aneglakya, devil's trumpet, hoh-eep, Indian apple, Jamestown weed, moh-mope, sacred datura, tolache.

PLANT DESCRIPTION: A perennial growing to 3 feet in height. The leaves are 2 inches long; the flowers, trumpet-shaped, erect, 7 to 8 inches long, white with purple markings; the capsule, 2 inches long, spined.

WHERE IT GROWS: Open fields, road-sides, prairie. Southern California, Arizona, New Mexico, and Texas.

WHAT IS HARVESTED AND WHEN: Leaves, roots, and seeds, as available and as needed.

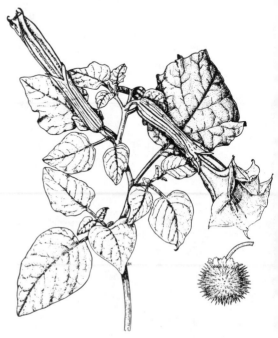

USES: Western Indians have used the bruised leaves and roots mixed with water as a narcotic and intoxicating drink. For the same purpose they have fermented the bruised seeds in water. The leaves have been smoked to cure shortness of breath. Poultices of mashed roots or mashed leaves were applied to burns, bruises, wounds, and cuts. An ointment made of mashed seeds and grease was applied to treat sores, boils, pimples, and swellings.

Datura stramonium L.

OTHER COMMON NAMES: apple of Peru, apple Peru, devil's apple, devil's trumpet, Jamestown weed, Jimsonweed datura, mad apple, stink apple, stinkweed, stinkwort, stramonium, thorn apple.

PLANT DESCRIPTION: An erect annual that grows to 4 feet in height. The leaves are 4 to 6 inches long, broad and unevenly toothed. The flowers are almost trumpet-shaped, pale blue. The plant produces large, prickly capsules filled with shiny black seeds.

WHERE IT GROWS: Throughout the United States in a wide range of habitats.

WHAT IS HARVESTED AND WHEN: Leaves, flowers, at maturity; roots, in the fall.

USES: This plant is a dangerous hallucinogen used by western Indians to induce visions. In Appalachia, a poultice made of the blossoms is applied to wounds to reduce pain. The dried leaves are smoked in a pipe or homemade cigarette to treat asthma. The leaves have also been applied to boils and ulcers. The pounded root has been used on wounds, bruises, and cuts. A decoction of blossoms and roots has been used as a sedative to calm patients during the setting of fractures. A treatment for asthma used by the pioneers was the inhaling of burning-leaf smoke—a procedure, legend tells us,

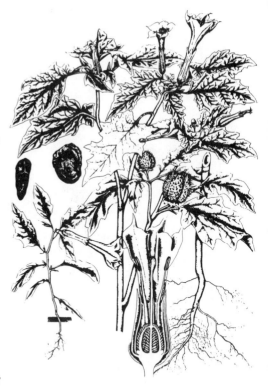

that was used by the Delphic Oracle to assist in divining the future.

WILD CARROT 89

Daucus carota L.

OTHER COMMON NAMES: bee's nest plant, bird's nest, bird's nest root, carrot, devil's plague, Queen Anne's lace.

PLANT DESCRIPTION: An erect, branching, fuzzy herb, 1 to 3 feet in height, biennial or perennial, arising from a thick, fleshy root. The leaves are pinnately divided. The flowers are white, cream, or yellow, borne in clusters, with a leaflike structure under each group of

flowers. The fruit is oblong, about 1/8 inch long, with some bristles.

WHERE IT GROWS: Open fields, waste places, and roadsides. Throughout the United States.

WHAT IS HARVESTED AND WHEN: Mature seeds, fruits, in late summer; roots, after the growing season.

USES: An infusion of the seeds and roots has been used to increase urine flow. The boiled mashed root has been applied as a poultice for bruises and cuts. The fruit has been eaten to stimulate menstruation; the seeds to treat intestinal worms.

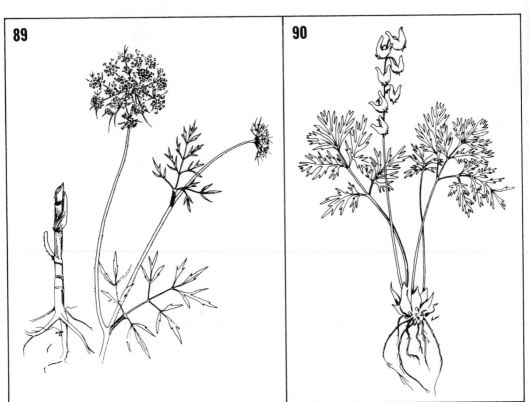

89

90

DUTCHMAN'S BREECHES 90

Dicentra cucullaria (L.) Bernh.

OTHER COMMON NAMES: breeches-flower, colicweed, little boy's breeches, little staggerweed, squirrel corn, turkey corn, white hearts.

PLANT DESCRIPTION: A perennial arising from a bulb and growing to 15 inches in height. The flowers are white or cream-colored. A close relative, **D.** canadensis (Goldie) Walp., has greenish white flowers with pink markings, and is aromatic.

WHERE IT GROWS: Rich, moist woods. New England to the Dakotas; south to Kansas, Georgia, Alabama, Mississippi, Missouri, North Carolina, and Tennessee; Washington and Oregon.

WHAT IS HARVESTED AND WHEN:
Underground parts, resembling peas or corn, in spring or fall.

USES: At one time the plant was substituted for mercury compounds in the treatment of venereal diseases. It has been used to increase urine flow, and as a tonic. A poultice has been used to treat skin diseases. Veterinarians have used it as a pre-anesthetic for larger animals.

COMMON FOXGLOVE   91

Digitalis purpurea L.

OTHER COMMON NAME: European foxglove.

PLANT DESCRIPTION: A biennial soft, fuzzy plant that grows to 4 feet in height. During the second summer of growth, a single erect stem arises from a leaf rosette and terminates in a group of large purple flowers that droop down.

WHERE IT GROWS: It is cultivated for drug use in Pennsylvania and grown in many states as an ornamental plant. A native of Europe, it has spread from New York to South Carolina, and is found in the West Coast states.

WHAT IS HARVESTED AND WHEN:
Leaves from first-year plants and second-year plants, as they begin to flower; seeds as they appear.

USES: The principal use of digitalis is as a heart stimulant, in the United States and elsewhere. Its medicinal value was known in England as far back as 1000 A.D.

It has also been used for neuralgia, insanity, heart palpitations, fever, and asthma.

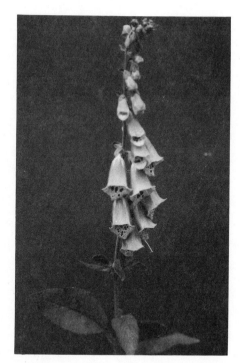

ATLANTIC YAM   92

Dioscorea villosa L.

OTHER COMMON NAMES: China root, colicroot, devil's bones, dioscorea, rheumatism root, wild gum root, wild yam, yam.

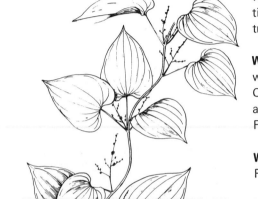

PLANT DESCRIPTION: A perennial vine that grows to 20 feet in length. The tiny flowers are green; the fruit is a triangular capsule.

WHERE IT GROWS: Roadsides, swamps, wet thickets, and hardwood forests. Connecticut and New York to Minnesota and Kansas; south to South Carolina, Florida, and Texas.

WHAT IS HARVESTED AND WHEN: Roots, in the fall; plant, at full bloom.

USES: Indians used a root decoction to relieve the pains of childbirth. The dried powdered root, boiled in water, was used to treat indigestion. Slaves used the root to treat muscular rheumatism. Taken internally, it has been used for muscle spasms, croup, gas, liver troubles, asthma, as a uterine tonic, and to induce vomiting. The plant itself is considered useful to release phlegm, induce vomiting, and increase urine flow.

PERSIMMON   93

Diospyros virginiana L.

OTHER COMMON NAMES: common persimmon, date plum, eastern persimmon, plaqueminier, possumwood, seeded plum, simmon, winter plum.

PLANT DESCRIPTION: A tree growing to 50 feet in height. The leaves are thick and firm, dark green above, paler and fuzzy below, 4 to 6 inches long, 1½ to 3 inches wide. The bark is thick, dark gray or brown, and prominently broken into square scaly areas. The flowers are greenish yellow to creamy white. The fruit is 1 to 1½ inches in diameter, yellow or orange, with flower sepals attached.

WHERE IT GROWS: Clearings, dry woods, and abandoned fields. Connecticut and Long Island along the coast to Florida; inland from Pennsylvania, Ohio, Indiana, and Illinois to Iowa; south through Kansas and Oklahoma to Texas.

WHAT IS HARVESTED AND WHEN:

Green fruits, in early fall; ripe fruits, after the first frost; roots, as needed.

USES: An infusion of the green fruit is used in treating diarrhea, dysentery, and uterine hemorrhages and as a gargle for sore throat. A drink made of powdered seeds mixed with water and strained through a cloth is used to treat kidney stones. Indians boiled the roots to make a medicinal tea for dysentery. They also washed babies mouths with an infusion of the boiled bark, as a remedy for sores on the mouth, lips, and throat.

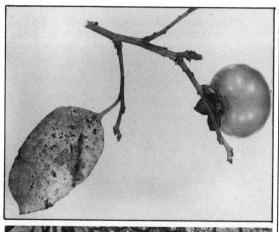

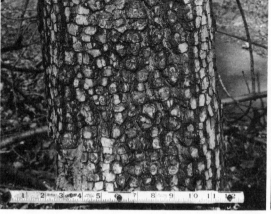

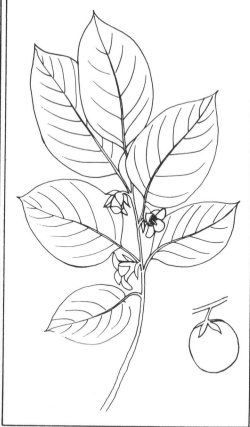

CRESTED FIELD FERN 94

Dryopteris cristata (L.) Gray

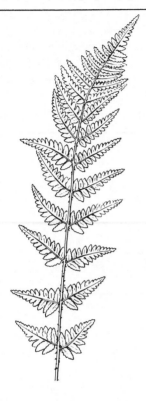

OTHER COMMON NAME: shield fern.

PLANT DESCRIPTION: A fern with stiff, erect fronds, growing to 2 feet in height. The reproductive bodies are found on the undersides of the fronds halfway between midrib and margins.

WHERE IT GROWS: Bogs, swamps, wet woods, thickets. New England south to the Appalachian highlands, North Carolina, and Louisiana; west to Ohio, Indiana, Missouri, and Nebraska.

WHAT IS HARVESTED AND WHEN: Roots, dug during the summer, then sliced and dried.

USES: The roots have been used to clear phlegm from the chest and to induce perspiring to break a fever, also as a treatment for intestinal worms.

MAYWEED DOGWEED 95

Dyssodia papposa (Vent.) Hitchc.

OTHER COMMON NAMES: fetid marigold, paugu'e.

PLANT DESCRIPTION: A strongly scented annual or biennial growing to 2 feet in height. The flowers are yellow.

WHERE IT GROWS: Hillsides and mountainsides, roadsides, and abandoned areas. Louisiana west to Arizona; north to Minnesota, Montana, North Dakota, and Illinois; east to New England.

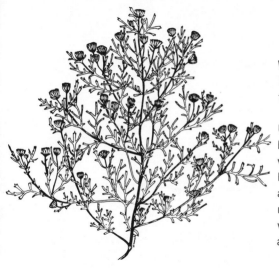

WHAT IS HARVESTED AND WHEN:
Leaves, when mature and large; seeds, as
they appear.

USES: A tea made of boiled fresh leaves
has been used to settle the stomach, stop
vomiting, and treat diarrhea. The fresh
leaves have been chewed to treat stomachache. For severe stomach colic, a liquid
made by soaking seeds in warm water
was given to babies. The fresh plant
applied to the skin can cause blisters.

PURPLE ECHINACEA   96

Echinacea purpurea (L.) Moench.

OTHER COMMON NAMES: black Samp-
son, comb-flower, hedgehog, purple cone
flower, red sunflower.

PLANT DESCRIPTION: A perennial
from 2 to 5 feet in height, with alternate
leaves, lance-shaped. Sometimes the base
of the leaf is winged; leaf margins are
toothed; top leaves lack stems. The flower
heads vary from purple to white.

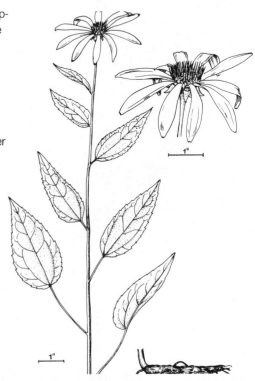

WHERE IT GROWS: Prairies, road
banks, and dry, open woods. Ohio to
Iowa, south to Oklahoma, Georgia, and
Alabama.

WHAT IS HARVESTED AND WHEN:
Roots, in the fall.

USES: It has been used medicinally for
rabies, syphilis, snakebite, skin diseases,
and blood poisoning.

Echinocereus enneacanthus Engelm.

OTHER COMMON NAME: pitahaya.

PLANT DESCRIPTION: A cactus with a cylindrical body, 6 inches high. The spines are straight; the flowers reddish purple, 4 inches long. The fruits are about 1 inch long and edible.

WHERE IT GROWS: At lower elevations in desert areas with low rainfall. Texas, New Mexico, and Arizona.

WHAT IS HARVESTED AND WHEN: Blossoms, in the spring.

USES: The flowers have been used to treat intestinal worms and to poison fish. New Mexicans use the blossoms in a tea to treat excessive water retention in the body.

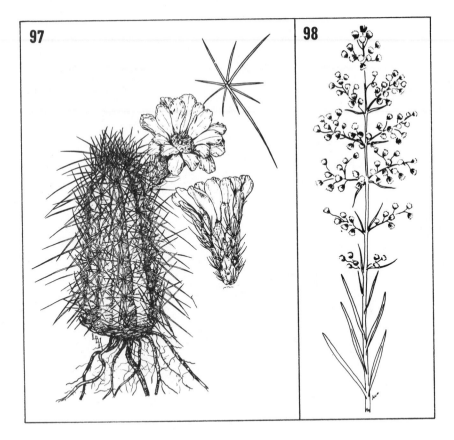

HORSEWEED   98

Erigeron canadensis L.

OTHER COMMON NAMES: bittersweet, bitterweed, bloodstaunch, butterweed, buttonweed, Canada erigeron, Canadian fleabane, colt's tail, cow's tail, fleabane, hogweed, mare's tail, pride weed.

PLANT DESCRIPTION: An annual growing to 6 feet in height. The leaves have bristles, and are sometimes toothed. The flowers range from white to purple.

WHERE IT GROWS: Old fields and pastures, empty lots. Throughout the United States.

WHAT IS HARVESTED AND WHEN: Leaves, when mature; tops, when in bloom.

USES: Indians made a decoction of the top leaves to treat dysentery, and early settlers adopted this practice. Indians also used the tops in their sauna baths, sprinkling them on the hot rocks. An oil obtained by distilling the plant has been used to treat diarrhea, hemorrhoids, and pulmonary problems. A decoction of the upper part of the plant has been used for sore throat.

STORK'S BILL   99

Erodium cicutarium (L.) L'Her.

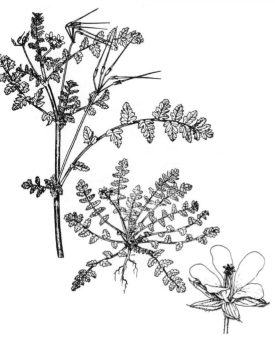

OTHER COMMON NAMES: alfilaria, common stork's bill, nenn's bill, pin clover, pin grass, pink needle, pin weed, red-stem filace.

PLANT DESCRIPTION: An annual or biennial, hairy, with rosettes during the winter. The leaflets lack stems. The flowers are rose to purple.

WHERE IT GROWS: Fields, roadsides, cultivated fields, waste places; cultivated in gardens. New England to Illinois and Michigan; south to Tennessee, North Carolina, Virginia, and Arkansas; west to Texas, New Mexico, Utah, and the Pacific Coast.

WHAT IS HARVESTED AND WHEN: Plants, when in bloom; leaves, when mature.

USES: The entire plant may be put into a warm-water bath for a person suffering the pains of rheumatism. The leaves have been made into a hot tea used to increase urine flow, to treat uterine hemorrhage and water retention, and to increase perspiration.

BUTTON'S SNAKEROOT ERYNGO   100

Eryngium aquaticum L.

OTHER COMMON NAMES: button snakeroot, corn snakeroot, eryngo, feverweed, rattlesnake flag, rattlesnake master, rattlesnake weed, water eryngo.

PLANT DESCRIPTION: An erect perennial that grows to 5 feet in height. The

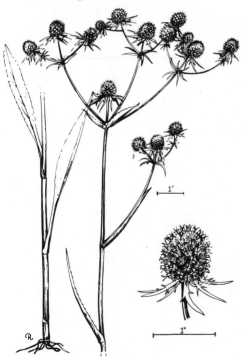

leaves are from 6 inches to 2 feet in length, and the upper ones have no stalks. The flowers are white and inconspicuous.

WHERE IT GROWS: Ponds and bogs, marshes, streams, and wet pinelands. New Jersey to Florida and Georgia, west to Texas.

WHAT IS HARVESTED AND WHEN: Rootstocks, in the fall; plants and stems, when in full bloom.

USES: Indians used this plant to prevent poisoning, reduce fever, and increase urine flow. They pounded the root, mixed it with water, and drank the potion as a cure for kidney trouble, neuralgia, and arthritis, and as a blood purifier. They also chewed the stems and leaves as a nosebleed remedy, and used a tea of the plants to cure severe dysentery. A decoction of the plant was drunk at some Indian ceremonials to induce vomiting. A decoction of the root was believed useful in treating kidney stone, laryngitis, gonorrhea, exhaustion from sexual depletion, and loss of erectile power.

BUTTON-SNAKEROOT   101

Eryngium yuccifolium Michx.

OTHER COMMON NAMES: rattlesnake master, yuccaleaf eryngo.

PLANT DESCRIPTION: An erect perennial growing to 5 feet in height. The leaves are long and narrow, up to 24 inches long, and 1 inch wide. The flowers are small, whitish to pale blue.

WHERE IT GROWS: Woods, old fields, prairies, and forested areas. New Jersey and Connecticut west to Ohio, Wisconsin, Michigan, and Minnesota, south to Kansas, and along the Atlantic coast to Georgia.

WHAT IS HARVESTED AND WHEN: Roots, as needed.

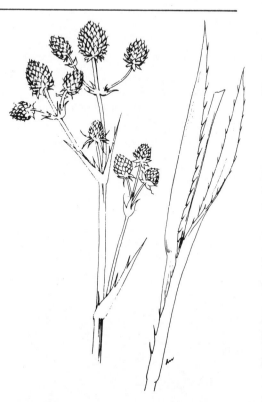

USES: The roots have been used medicinally for liver ailments, to increase urine flow, to induce vomiting, and to treat rattlesnake bite. Chewing the root results in increased saliva flow. A liquid made from roots mashed in cold water was drunk to relieve muscular pains. The roots have also been used for rheumatism, respiratory ailments, and kidney trouble, and to increase perspiration. Indians used them for bladder problems.

CORALBEAD   102

Erythrina herbacea L.

OTHER COMMON NAME: eastern coralbean.

PLANT DESCRIPTION: A shrub with stems growing to 5 feet in height, sometimes a tree up to 25 feet high in the southern United States. The leaves have prickly stems and three leaflets, occasionally prickly beneath. The flowers are 2 inches long, dark red; the pods about 5 inches long; the seeds, bright red with black spots.

WHERE IT GROWS: Open sandy woods, glades, and clearings. North Carolina to Florida, Mississippi, and Texas.

WHAT IS HARVESTED AND WHEN:
Seeds, when mature; plants, in full bloom; roots, as needed.

USES: Decoctions of the plant have been used in the Southwest as a laxative and to increase urine flow and perspiration. Indians ate the roots to increase perspiration. The beans have been used to poison rats and render animals inactive, somewhat as curare is used to paralyze fish in South America.

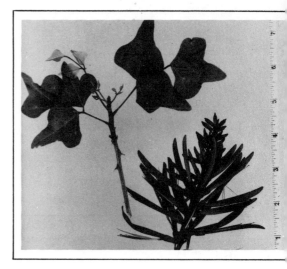

YELLOW FAWN LILY   103

Erythronium grandiflorum Pursh.

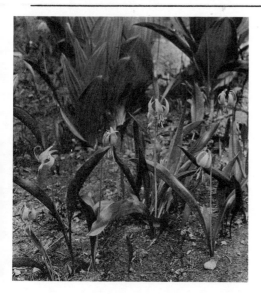

PLANT DESCRIPTION: A low, short-stemmed perennial, with two leaves arising from the base and golden yellow flowers.

WHERE IT GROWS: Open pine forests, cutover lands, and prairies. Washington, Oregon, and northern California to Nevada, Utah, western Colorado, and western Montana.

WHAT IS HARVESTED AND WHEN:
Underground bulbs, in the fall or in the second year of growth or later.

USES: Indians crushed the bulbs to make a poultice for treating boils. They believed that a wash made of the bulbs cooked in water would protect them from snakebites.

OTHER COMMON NAME: Dog-toothed violet.

FEVERTREE 104

Eucalyptus globulus Labill.

OTHER COMMON NAMES: blue gum, Tasmanian blue eucalyptus, Tasmanian blue gum.

PLANT DESCRIPTION: A tall tree growing to 300 feet in height. The bark peels in long strips or sheets from the smooth gray or bluish trunk. The fruit is 1½ inches wide.

WHERE IT GROWS: As a cultivated plant in California.

WHAT IS HARVESTED AND WHEN: Bark, roots, and leaves, as needed.

USES: The leaves are distilled to produce eucalyptol, which is used internally to treat bronchitis, tuberculosis, and nose and throat inflammations. Vapor made by boiling the leaves, bark, or roots, or distilling them in water has been used as an inhalant for diphtheria, coughs, and respiratory ailments. Leaf poultices have been used to bring abscesses to a head. The leaves have been prepared for internal use to treat intestinal worms.

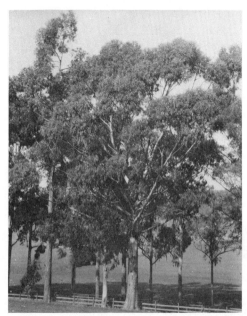

WAHOO 105

Euonymus americanus L.

OTHER COMMON NAMES: arrowwood, burning-bush, bursting heart, fishwood, spindle tree, strawberry bush, strawberry tree.

PLANT DESCRIPTION: A shrub growing to 6 feet in height. The leaves have short stalks and are bright green, 1½ to 3 inches long, and ½ to 1¼ inches wide. The flowers are small, greenish in color, and 1/3 inch long.

WHERE IT GROWS: Ravines, stream banks, rocky places, and damp glades. New York to Florida and Texas.

WHAT IS HARVESTED AND WHEN: Bark and roots, in spring or fall; seeds, in the fall.

USES: The powdered bark has been used as a remedy for dandruff and scalp irritation. The bark of the root has been prepared for internal use as a laxative, to reduce fever, and to increase urine flow. A decoction of the bark has been taken to treat uterine troubles, venereal diseases, and skin ailments and to induce vomiting. The seeds have been used as a strong laxative.

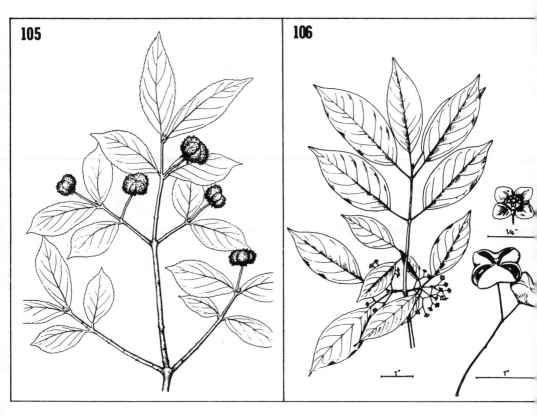

EASTERN WAHOO   106

Euonymus atropurpureus Jacq.

OTHER COMMON NAMES: American spindle tree, arrow-wood, bitter ash, bleeding heart, bursting heart, Indian arrow-wood, pegwood, prickwood, purple strawberry bush, sindle tree, skewerwood, spindle tree, strawberry bush, wahoo.

PLANT DESCRIPTION: A shrub or small tree that grows to 25 feet in height. It has green branches and purplish flowers. The fruit is bright red and four-lobed.

WHERE IT GROWS: Damp forests and thickets, swamps, and stream banks. New York to Florida and Texas, west to Montana and Oklahoma.

WHAT IS HARVESTED AND WHEN: Root bark and stem bark, as needed; seeds, in the fall.

USES: Indian women drank a decoction of the inner-stem bark for uterine discomfort and used the same preparation as an eye lotion. A poultice of pounded stem bark or root bark was applied to facial sores. The pioneers used the bark as a liver stimulant and a laxative, and for fever and indigestion. It was also used in the treatment of secondary syphilis. An oil from the seed was used, both in Europe and the United States, to destroy head lice.

BONESET   107

Eupatorium perfoliatum L.

OTHER COMMON NAMES: ague-weed, common boneset, crosswort, feverwort, Indian sage, Joepye, sweating plant, sweating weed, teagel, thoroughstem, thoroughwax, thoroughwort, throughstem, vegetable antimony, wild Isaac, wild sage.

PLANT DESCRIPTION: A perennial bush that grows to 5 feet in height, with heavy, slightly hairy stems and opposite leaves. The flowers are purplish to white, borne in flat heads.

WHERE IT GROWS: Damp, moist areas such as swamps, rich woods, marshes, pastures, and prairies. New England and New York, south to Florida, Alabama, and Louisiana, and west to Texas and the Dakotas.

WHAT IS HARVESTED AND WHEN: Entire plant, in early spring when full-grown; leaves and flowering tops (without larger, coarser stems), in late summer.

USES: In Appalachia, a tea made from the leaves is used as a laxative and as a

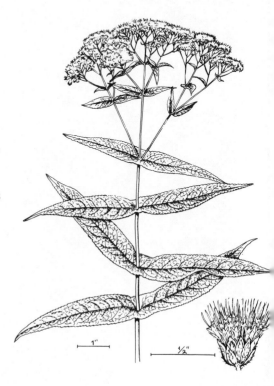

treatment for coughs and chest illnesses. In the last century, boneset tea was widely used as a remedy for colds and coughs. Indian women who complained of aches and pains were given a steam treatment—inhalation of the vapors from boiling plants. Negro slaves and Indians used the plant to treat malarial fever. Confederate Army surgeons prescribed it as a treatment for worms.

SWEET JOE-PYE-WEED   108

Eupatorium purpureum L.

OTHER COMMON NAMES: green-stemmed joe-pye weed, hemp weed, Jopi-root, kidney root, purple boneset, Queen of the Meadow, thoroughwort.

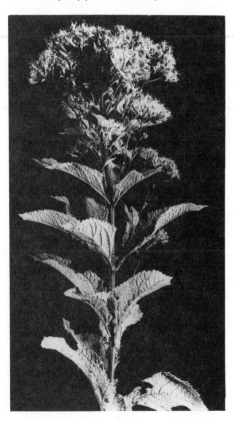

PLANT DESCRIPTION: A perennial with hollow stems growing to 10 feet in height. The whorled leaves, 4 to 6 in a whorl, are 4 to 12 inches long and coarsely toothed. The flowers are purple.

WHERE IT GROWS: Rich dry to moist woods, waste places, old fields, along banks of streams, and swampy areas. New England to Minnesota, Nebraska, Oklahoma, and Arkansas, south to Florida.

WHAT IS HARVESTED AND WHEN: Entire plant, in full bloom; roots, in the fall.

USES: Indians used the plant to induce sweating and break a fever. Pioneers used it for the same purpose in treating typhus fever, as well as to induce vomiting and for bladder ailments. As an internal remedy, the root has been administered to increase urine flow, for urinary infections and female disorders, and as a tonic and a stimulant.

Euphorbia maculata L.

OTHER COMMON NAMES: black scourge, bowman's root, emetic weed, eyebane, milk purslane; spotted euphorbia, wort weed, yerba de la golondrina.

PLANT DESCRIPTION: A flat annual whose stems form a mat. The leaves are ½ inch long, slightly toothed near the apex, often with a red spot. The plant exudes a milky sap when crushed.

WHERE IT GROWS: In dry, open soil on woodsides, in fields, lawns, gardens, and meadows. New England and New York, west to Michigan, Wisconsin, Minnesota, the Dakotas, Wyoming, and California, south to Florida and Texas.

WHAT IS HARVESTED AND WHEN: Plant (for juice) and roots, during the growing season.

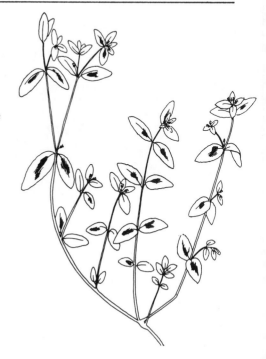

USES: The milky sap, when taken orally, causes vomiting and acts as a strong laxative. An alcoholic extract of the plant has been given to control dysentery. The Indians rubbed the sap on their skin to treat warts, sores, eruptions, and sore nipples. They also drank a root infusion as a laxative.

Fagus grandifolia Ehrh.

OTHER COMMON NAMES: American beech, red beech, ridge beech, stone beech, white beech, winter beech.

PLANT DESCRIPTION: A tree growing to 100 feet in height. The leaves are 2 to 5 inches long, silky when immature, bluish green above, turning bright yellow in autumn. The fruit is about ¾ inch long, with prickles.

WHERE IT GROWS: Rich, moist soils, and in coastal plains areas. New England to Massachusetts, Ohio, Illinois, and Mis-

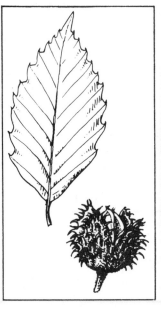 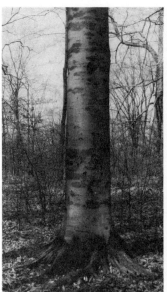 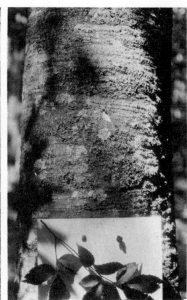

souri; south to West Virginia, Virginia, and Florida; west to Texas.

WHAT IS HARVESTED AND WHEN: Leaves, when mature; bark, as needed.

USES: A concoction made of fresh or dried leaves was applied by the pioneers to burns, scalds, and frostbite. Indians steeped a handful of fresh bark in a cup or two of water and used it for skin rashes, particularly those caused by poison ivy.

VIRGINIA STRAWBERRY   111

Fragaria virginiana Duchesne

OTHER COMMON NAMES: alpine strawberry, Indian strawberry, scarlet strawberry, strawberry, wild strawberry.

PLANT DESCRIPTION: A low-running perennial with three leaflets. The flowers have five white petals, and the fruit is a small strawberry.

WHERE IT GROWS: Open slopes, fields, lawn edges, and borders of woods. New England south to Georgia, Tennessee, the Carolinas, and Appalachia, and west to Oklahoma.

WHAT IS HARVESTED AND WHEN: Leaves and fruit, when large enough; roots, in the fall.

USES: The berries were once thought helpful in treating kidney stones and gout. An infusion of the root has been used in England for gonorrhea. A tea made from the leaves has been used to treat diarrhea. The roots have been considered excellent as bitters to increase urine flow.

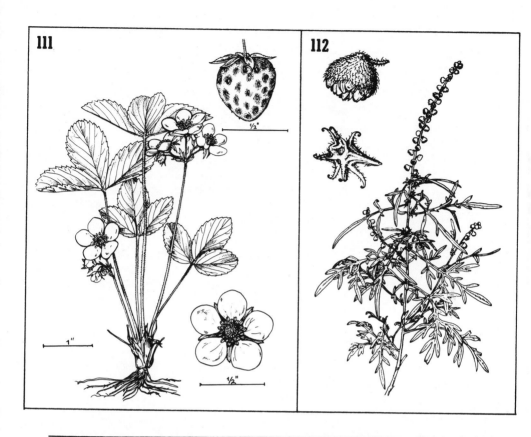

TOAD HERB   112

Franseria tenuifolia Harv. and Gray

PLANT DESCRIPTION: A woody perennial growing to 2 feet in height. The stems are covered with long, spreading white hairs. The leaves are over 2 inches long. The fruits have a single beak and hooked spines.

WHERE IT GROWS: Sandy soils at higher elevations. New Mexico, Texas, Arizona, and California.

WHAT IS HARVESTED AND WHEN: Roots, in the fall; leaves, when mature.

USES: The ground-up root has been placed in tooth cavities to relieve toothache. A tea made of the leaves—either green or dried and ground—has been used for stomach distress.

Fraxinus americana L.

OTHER COMMON NAMES: American ash, American white ash, ash, biltmore ash, biltmore white ash, cane ash, smallseed white ash.

PLANT DESCRIPTION: A tree that may grow to 120 feet in height. The bark is ashy gray and furrowed. The leaves are 8 to 12 inches long, with five to nine (mostly 7) leaflets 3 to 5 inches long, rounded at the base, and half as wide as they are long. The winged seeds are 1 to 3 inches long, narrow and flat, and occur in clusters.

WHERE IT GROWS: Rich, rather moist soils on low hills and near streams, in upland to lowland woods. All eastern states, including northern Florida.

WHAT IS HARVESTED AND WHEN: Inner bark of trunk and roots, and stems of branches, in spring or fall; leaves, any time during the growing season; seeds, in late summer and early fall.

USES: In Appalachia, the chewed bark is applied on sores as a poultice. A tea made from the buds is thought useful for snakebite—a belief shared by early Indians. Another belief was that the seeds were aphrodisiac and also increased the appetite and urine flow. Indians made a strong tea from the leaves and gave it to women after childbirth. The bark, taken internally, was supposed to increase perspiration and urine flow.

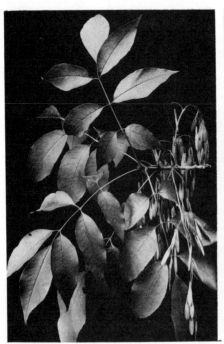
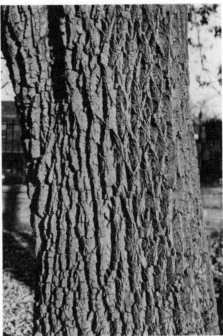

Galium aparine L.

OTHER COMMON NAMES: bedstraw, catchweed, cheese rennet herb, chicus, clabber-grass, cleavers, cleaver's herb, cleaves, cleverwort, goosegrass, goose's hare, milksweet, poor robin, savoyan, scratchweed, spring cleavers, turkey grass.

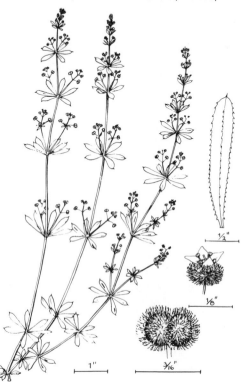

PLANT DESCRIPTION: An annual plant that has a weak, reclining, bristly four-angled stem with hairy joints. The leaves occur in whorls of eight. The flowers are white, borne in a broad, flat cluster. The fruits are very bristly.

WHERE IT GROWS: Rich woods, thickets, seashores, waste ground, and shady areas. Canada to Florida and west to Texas.

WHAT IS HARVESTED AND WHEN: Entire plant, during flowering in mid-summer.

USES: This plant has been used to increase urine flow, to stimulate the appetite, to reduce fever, and to remedy vitamin C deficiency. It has also been used as a wash to remove freckles.

Gaultheria procumbens L.

OTHER COMMON NAMES: aromatic wintergreen, berried tea, boxberry, Canadian tea, checkerberry, chequerberry, chickerberry, clink, creeping wintergreen, deerberry, dewberry, ground holly, ground ivy, grouse berry, hillberry, ivory plum, mountain berry, mountain tea, mountain teaberry, partridge berry, pigeonberry, red-berry tea, red pollom, roxberry, spice berry, spicy wintergreen, spring wintergreen, teaberry, three-leaved wintergreen, trailing gaultheria, wax cluster, winterberry, wintergreen.

PLANT DESCRIPTION: A low, creeping, aromatic evergreen shrub, with 2- to 6-

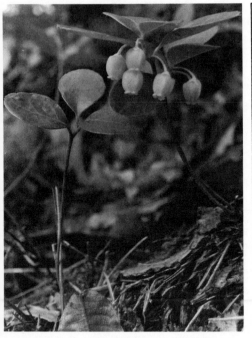

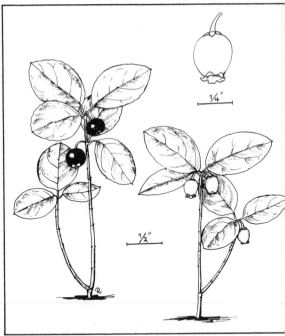

inch branches. The leaves are shiny and waxy, and the single white, nodding flowers occur in leaf axils. The plant produces bright red berries in fall and winter.

WHERE IT GROWS: Dry, wooded areas, sterile woods, and clearings, generally found growing with rhododendron and mountain laurel. North Carolina, Virginia, Kentucky, and West Virginia.

WHAT IS HARVESTED AND WHEN: Leaves, as needed; whole plant, when in full bloom.

USES: A tea made from the leaves has been used to relieve pain and treat rheumatism. The plant has also been used to treat dysentery and bring on delayed menstruation, to promote milk flow in nursing mothers, and as a cure for toothache. The plant is the source of wintergreen oil, which is used as a flavoring, as a counterirritant to relieve gas and colic, and to reduce the swelling of tissues.

VELVETWEED 116

Gaura parviflora Dougl.

PLANT DESCRIPTION: A single-stemmed, hairy annual or biennial that grows to 6 feet in height. The soft, hairy leaves, 2 to 4 inches long, first form a ground rosette. The small, reddish flowers, with four petals ½ inch long, are stalkless and crowded on a spike at the top of the plant.

106

WHERE IT GROWS: Old fields, road-sides, overgrazed pastures, high desert grasslands, and sandy river plains, from 100 to 7,000 feet elevation. Louisiana to Arizona, north to Washington and west to South Dakota.

WHAT IS HARVESTED AND WHEN: Entire plant, when in bloom.

USES: A poultice made of the crushed plant has been used to treat muscular pains and arthritis.

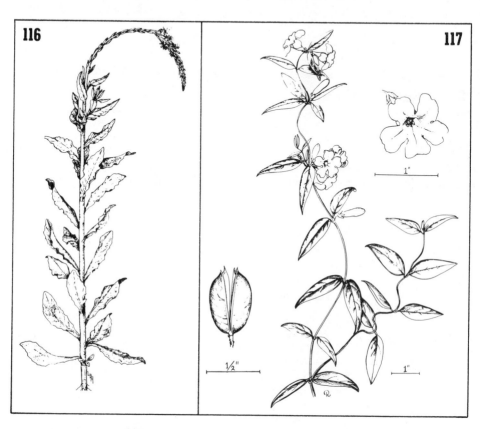

YELLOW JESSAMINE 117

Gelsemium sempervirens (L.) Ait.

OTHER COMMON NAMES: Carolina jessamine, evening trumpet flower, false jasmine, false jessamine, gelsemium, jasmine, wild jasmine, wild jessamine, woodbine, yellow jasmine root.

PLANT DESCRIPTION: A perennial vine with a horizontal, branched, cylin-drical rootstock that is brown to yellow

orange and has a peculiar odor. The leaves are short-stalked, lance-shaped, aromatic, and evergreen, with smooth margins. The flowers are yellow, showy, fragrant, and tube-shaped.

WHERE IT GROWS: Thickets, dry and wet woods, fence rows, edges of woods, and stream banks; trailing on the ground or climbing trees, bushes, or fences. Florida west to Texas, north to Virginia, Tennessee, and Arkansas.

WHAT IS HARVESTED AND WHEN:
Roots and rhizomes, in spring or just after flowering in late summer; flowers, as they appear.

USES: A tea made of the flowers was once thought to be good for coughs, shortness of breath, pleurisy, and stomach pains, as well as to help in childbirth. Preparations made from the roots and rhizomes have been used as a central nervous system depressant, to reduce fever, and to relieve pain.

SAMPSON'S SNAKEROOT   118

Gentiana villosa L.

OTHER COMMON NAMES: marsh gentian, straw-colored gentian, striped gentian.

PLANT DESCRIPTION: A perénnial with several smooth, ascending stems. The leaves are lance-shaped. A cluster of crowded, tubular, greenish white to purplish green flowers grows at the top of the plant.

WHERE IT GROWS: Meadows, brook sides, slopes, calcareous rocks, woods, and pinelands. Florida west to Louisiana, north to New Jersey, Pennsylvania, Ohio, and Indiana

WHAT IS HARVESTED AND WHEN:
Rhizomes and roots, in the fall.

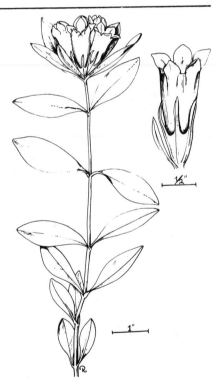

USES: In Appalachia, a root tea is drunk as a tonic, and a piece of the rhizome is sometimes worn or carried in the belief that it will increase one's physical powers. The rhizome has been used to treat indigestion, gout, and rheumatism and to reduce vomiting. It has been used as a tonic, as an aid to digestion, for nervous distress, and for gout.

Geranium maculatum L.

OTHER COMMON NAMES: alum bloom, alumroot, American kind, American tormentil, astringent root, chocolate flower, common crane's bill, cranesbill, cranesbill geranium, crowfoot, dove's foot, old maid's nightcap, shame-face, spotted cranesbill, stork bill, tormentil, wild cranesbill, wild geranium.

PLANT DESCRIPTION: A perennial 1 to 2 feet in height, with a single stem and thick rhizomes. The leaves are 3 to 6 inches across, and deeply cleft. Each plant produces three to five loose, rosy-purple to white flowers 1 inch wide.

WHERE IT GROWS: In rich woods, thickets, and meadows and along fence rows. New England; south to Tennessee and Georgia; west to Missouri and Kansas

WHAT IS HARVESTED AND WHEN: Leaves and rhizomes, in spring just before flowering or in late summer.

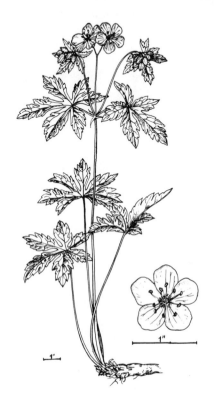

USES: In Appalachia, a tea made from the above-ground parts of the plant is used to treat dysentery and sore throat. The leaves have been used as a poultice to hasten the healing of open wounds: Indians used the powdered dried roots to stop bleeding from cuts, scratches, and wounds. The roots and rhizomes are considered antiseptic and have been used to increase urine flow, reduce swellings, and treat diarrhea.

Geum rivale L.

OTHER COMMON NAMES: bennet, chocolate-root, cureall, Evan's root, Indian chocolate, purple avens, throat root.

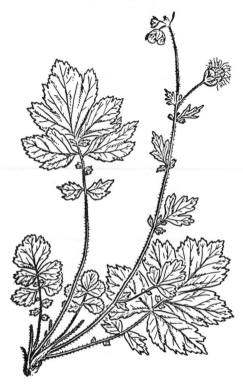

PLANT DESCRIPTION: A perennial plant with a basal rosette, growing to 4½ feet in height. The leaves, on the stem, are three-lobed. The flowers are purple or dark yellow.

WHERE IT GROWS: Damp and wet areas, bogs, highly organic soils, and cooler regions. New England to West Virginia and Ohio, Illinois, and Minnesota; as far west as New Mexico.

WHAT IS HARVESTED AND WHEN: Above-ground parts, in spring before blossoming; roots, as needed.

USES: Chopped and mixed with sugar and milk, the roots or tops have been taken internally for dysentery, indigestion, and rundown conditions. A root decoction has been used to treat hemorrhages, menstrual disorders, intestinal worms, and stomach ulcers.

INDIAN PHYSIC   121

Gillenia trifoliata (L.) Moench.

OTHER COMMON NAMES: American ipecac, Beaumont root, Bowman's root, false ipecac, Indian hippo, ipecacum, three-leaved spiraea, western dropwort.

PLANT DESCRIPTION: A perennial 2 to 4 feet in height, with slightly hairy, reddish stems. The flowers are white or pinkish, 1 inch across, with narrow petals.

WHERE IT GROWS: Rich woods at higher elevations. Delaware south along the Appalachian Mountains and the Atlantic Coast to the Carolinas, Georgia, and Alabama.

WHAT IS HARVESTED AND WHEN: Roots, in the fall.

USES: Large doses of the powdered dry root have been used to induce vomiting; smaller doses for a tonic. The root bark has been used to induce gentle vomiting and to treat rheumatism, dyspepsia, intestinal worms, and retention of water in the body. The dried root has been used as a strong laxative and tonic. Indians used it to cure fever and chronic diarrhea.

121

122

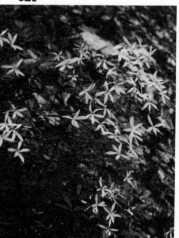

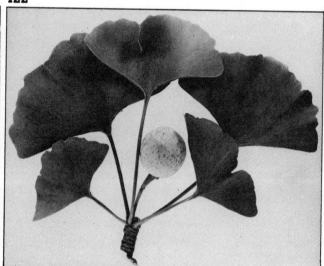

GINKGO   122

Ginkgo biloba L.

OTHER COMMON NAME: maidenhair tree.

PLANT DESCRIPTION: A tree that grows to over 100 feet in height, with fan-shaped leaves 2 to 4 inches across. The fruit is 1 inch long, yellow, and ill-smelling, with an edible sweet kernel, or nut, within.

WHERE IT GROWS: This remarkably adaptable cultivated tree, a native of China, grows well in suburban plantings and in cities, despite high pollution rates. It has been planted in many parts of the United States as far north as Ithaca, New York.

WHAT IS HARVESTED AND WHEN: Fruit and seeds, in the fall.

USES: The fruit has been used to treat bronchial complaints and gonorrhea, to soothe stomach distress, and to kill worms. As a poultice it has been applied to cuts and wounds. These nuts have been used to calm upset people and to release phlegm from the throat. The seeds are eaten in China.

Glycyrrhiza lepidota (Nutt.) Pursh.

OTHER COMMON NAMES: amalillo, American licorice.

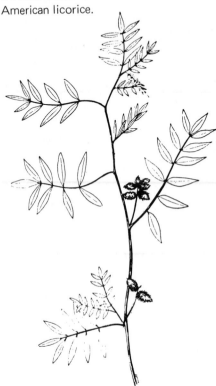

PLANT DESCRIPTION: An erect perennial growing to 3 feet in height. The flowers, pale yellow to white, appear at the end of flower stalks. The pods are brown, with hooks, resembling cockleburs.

WHERE IT GROWS: Prairies of the West, along railroad right-of-ways, and shores of lakes. Pacific Coast states through the Southwest, Midwest, and East.

WHAT IS HARVESTED AND WHEN: Roots from mature plants, in the fall.

USES: An extract of the roots has been included in cough mixtures to help bring up chest phlegm. Taken internally, wild licorice has been used to treat stomach ulcers, rheumatism, and arthritis. A root decoction has been used to induce menstrual flow, to treat fever in nursing mothers, and to facilitate the expelling of the afterbirth.

GUM PLANT   124

Grindelia squarrosa (Pursh.) Dunal.

OTHER COMMON NAMES: broad-leaved gumplant, curlcup gumweed, curlycup gumweed, rayless gumweed, resinweed, rosinweed, scaly grindelia, tarweed.

PLANT DESCRIPTION: A biennial or perennial growing to 3 feet in height. The leaves are toothed, 2½ inches long. The flowers are sticky, yellow, and 1½ inches across.

WHERE IT GROWS: Western plains and ranges, dry areas, and glades. Almost all states east of the Rockies.

WHAT IS HARVESTED AND WHEN: Leaves and flowering tops, as needed; roots, in the fall or spring.

USES: A decoction of the flowering tops and leaves was used to treat gonorrhea,

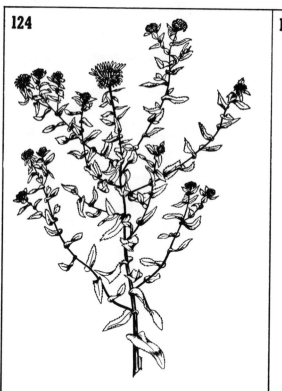

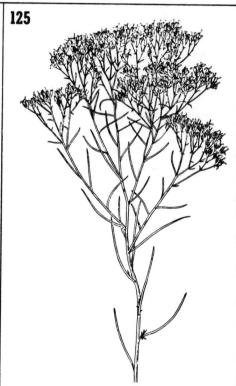

pneumonia, smallpox, and lung diseases. A tea of the same plant parts was administered to relieve stomachache and to treat urinary ailments and skin rashes from

toxic plants such as poison ivy. Indians made a tea of the root for liver trouble. A poultice of the plant was applied to rheumatic joints.

BROOM SNAKEROOT   125

Gutierrezia sarothrae (Pursh.) Britt. and Rusby

OTHER COMMON NAMES: broomweed, matchweed, snakeweed.

PLANT DESCRIPTION: A low, compact perennial shrub ½ to 2 feet in height. Its many slender and much-branched stems have woody bases. The leaves are slender, 3/8 to 1½ inches long, with smooth margins. The yellow, sticky flowers grow in dense clusters.

WHERE IT GROWS: This pest is found on open grasslands and woodland ranges, often associated with poor range management. It is found in a wide variety of soils, at elevations of 2,500 to 7,000 feet. Montana, Idaho, Wyoming, Utah, Arizona, Texas, Nevada, and California.

WHAT IS HARVESTED AND WHEN: Above-ground parts, at full bloom.

USES: A tea made of the plant has been used to treat stomachache and snakebites. A liquid remedy made by boiling the plants in water has been used as a rheumatism liniment and for malaria.

Hamamelis virginiana L.

OTHER COMMON NAMES: common witch hazel, hamamelis, long boughs, pistachio, snapping hazel, snapping hazelnut, southern witch hazel, spotted alder, striped alder, tobacco wood, white hazel, winterbloom, wood tobacco.

PLANT DESCRIPTION: A crooked tree or shrub 8 to 15 feet in height, with forking branches and smooth brown bark. The leaves are roundish to round-oval, 3 to 5 inches long, thick, and borne on a short stalk. Yellow, threadlike flowers appear in late fall or early winter after the leaves have fallen. The fruits grow in clusters along the stem and mature the following season, when they burst open and eject shiny black seeds.

WHERE IT GROWS: Dry to moist woods, usually on borders of forests, in rich soils, and on rocky banks of streams. New England to Georgia and Nebraska; northern Michigan and southern Minnesota south to Florida, Texas, Tennessee, and Missouri.

WHAT IS HARVESTED AND WHEN: Leaves, in summer or fall; twigs and bark, in spring or fall.

USES: The twigs, leaves, and bark are the basis of witch hazel extract, included in many medicinal lotions for bruises and sprains and in shaving lotions. Indians used this plant widely. They applied the bark to skin tumors and skin inflammations, used the inner bark as a poultice on irritated eyes, and chewed the bark to freshen their mouths. A boiled solution was rubbed on the legs of Indian athletes to keep them limber; it was also used to treat lame back. Another Indian custom was to place witch hazel twigs in water and add heated rocks to create a "sauna" for treating sore muscles. Distilled witch hazel extract has been used to treat hemorrhoids.

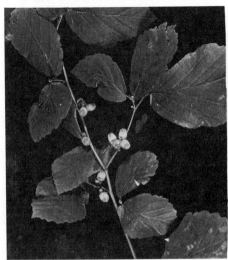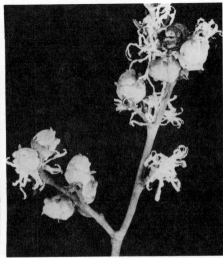

Hedeoma pulegioides (L.) Pers.

OTHER COMMON NAMES: American false-pennyroyal, mock pennyroyal, pennyroyal, Pennyroyal of America, pudding grass, squaw mint, stinking balm, thickweed, tickweed.

PLANT DESCRIPTION: A branched annual that grows to 18 inches in height. The leaves are erect, hairy, small, and ovate, with the broad end at the base. Aromatic tiny bluish flowers, about ¼ inch long are produced in clusters.

WHERE IT GROWS: Dry soils, woodlands, pastures, and meadows. Minnesota, South Dakota, and New England, south to Virginia, West Virginia, Florida, Mississippi, Louisiana, Tennessee, Kentucky, Arkansas, and Texas.

WHAT IS HARVESTED AND WHEN: Above-ground plant parts, at full bloom.

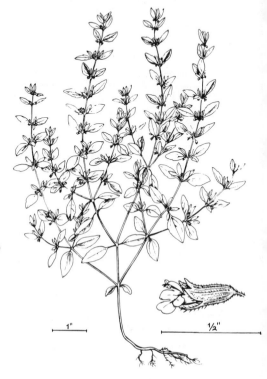

USES: A tea made of the above-ground parts of the plant is used in Appalachia for treating pneumonia. Indians used such a tea for headaches, and in colonial times it was recommended for delayed menstruation and to induce perspiration in people with bad colds. Boiled in water, the plant was used by Indians to relieve itching eyes. It is considered useful for reducing spasms and convulsions, and as a stimulant.

SNEEZEWEED   128

Helenium amarum (Raf.) H. Rock.

OTHER COMMON NAME: bitterweed.

PLANT DESCRIPTION: A perennial growing to 3 feet in height, with smooth lower leaves that are absent at flowering. The many yellow flowers occur on stalks 1 to 4 inches long.

WHERE IT GROWS: Dry glades, roadsides, old pastures, stream banks, open woods. Virginia and Tennessee south to Florida, Mississippi, and Alabama; west to Texas, Missouri, and Kansas.

WHAT IS HARVESTED AND WHEN: Entire plant, when in bloom.

USES: The plant has been used to cause sneezing and thus clear the nasal passages of mucus; also as a strong fish poison.

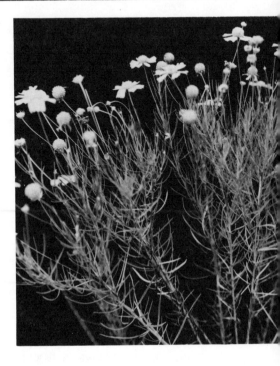

SNEEZEWEED   129

Helenium autumnale L.

OTHER COMMON NAME: bitterweed.

PLANT DESCRIPTION A perennial growing to 6 feet in height. The leaves are toothed, 3 to 5 inches long. The flowers are yellow.

WHERE IT GROWS: Old fields, meadows, and along the seashore. A number of varieties exist, and the plants are spread widely throughout the United States.

WHAT IS HARVESTED AND WHEN: Flowers, when mature; leaves, as needed.

USES: The flowers and leaves have been snuffed to cause sneezing and clear nasal passages, and to treat colds. The plant parts and flowers have been used to treat intestinal worms. They have been thought to be poisonous to fish and insects.

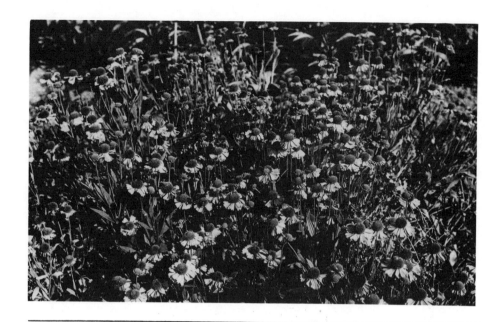

HERB-OF-THE-WOLF   130

Helenium hoopesii Gray

OTHER COMMON NAME: Yerba del lobo.

PLANT DESCRIPTION: A perennial 1 to 3 feet in height, with yellowish green leaves 4 to 10 inches long. The flowers are yellow, 3 inches in diameter, with drooping petals.

WHERE IT GROWS: At elevations from 7,500 to 11,000 feet in moist, well-drained meadows and the deep, rich soils of coniferous forests. Wyoming, New Mexico, Arizona, California, Rocky Mountains, and Oregon.

WHAT IS HARVESTED AND WHEN: Roots, from plants one year old or older.

USES: Pains due to rheumatism or pulmonary diseases are treated by rubbing with the dried, ground roots. A tea made by boiling the roots has been used to

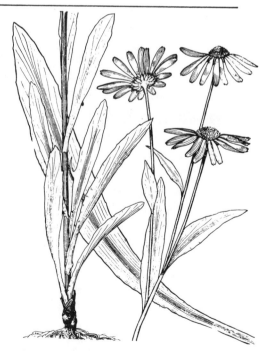

treat stomachache and diarrhea, and to eliminate intestinal worms.

ROCK ROSE   131

Helianthemum canadense (L.) Michx.

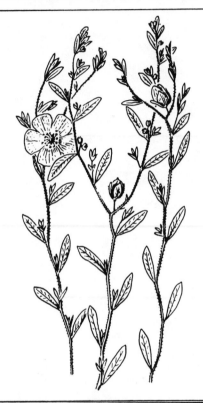

OTHER COMMON NAMES: frostweed, frostwort.

PLANT DESCRIPTION: A small perennial growing to 18 inches in height, hairy, with leaves about 1 inch long. The flowers are borne twice during the summer; they are bright yellow and shed their petals the day after full bloom.

WHERE IT GROWS: Dry, sandy soils, clearings, and open glades. New England south to North Carolina, Kentucky, and Tennessee; west to Missouri and Wisconsin.

WHAT IS HARVESTED AND WHEN: Entire plant, when in bloom.

USES: A decoction was used to treat diarrhea, syphilis, sore throat, and skin diseases.

COMMON SUNFLOWER   132

Helianthus annuus L.

PLANT DESCRIPTION: The plant may grow as high as 18 feet. The flower heads are conspicuous for their size and black and yellow color.

WHERE IT GROWS: Gardens, plains, old, abandoned fields, roadsides, rich, damp soils. Throughout the United States.

WHAT IS HARVESTED AND WHEN: Flowers, in summer; leaves, when mature.

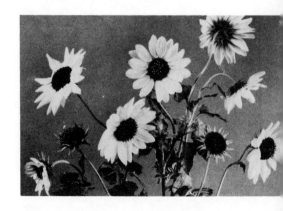

USES: In the last century, it was believed that a sunflower growing near a home would protect the family from malaria. At one time, an infusion of the flowers was used to kill flies. A warm bath containing either green or dried flowers was used by the early settlers to relieve rheumatism and other aches and pains. The plant parts have been considered effective in treating bronchitis and other respiratory troubles.

SUNFLOWER   133

Helianthus strumosus L.

OTHER COMMON NAME: soleil.

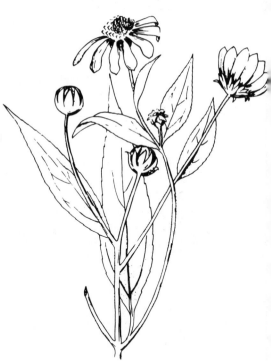

PLANT DESCRIPTION: An annual growing to 10 feet in height. The leaves are rough on the upper surface, pale green and fuzzy beneath. The flower is the familiar sunflower.

WHERE IT GROWS: Sunny, open woods and clearings. New England to North Dakota; south to Georgia and Alabama; west to Oklahoma and Arkansas.

WHAT IS HARVESTED AND WHEN: Seeds, when ripe; roots, at end of summer.

USES: The sunflower has many common uses. Indians applied the crushed root to bruises. The seeds have been used to increase urine flow and to clear phlegm. Many Indians ground them into meal and baked it for food.

SHARPLOBE HEPATICA   134

Hepatica acutiloba DC.

OTHER COMMON NAMES: heart liver-leaf, hepatica, liverleaf, liverwort, noble liverwort, sharplobed liverleaf.

PLANT DESCRIPTION: A perennial that grows to 9 inches in height. Its liver-shaped leaves have three to five lobes, and each leaf stalk has one leaf. A single white to purplish flower appears in spring.

WHERE IT GROWS: Rich, calcareous woods, mountains. Maine to Minnesota, Georgia to Alabama and Missouri, Tennessee, Kentucky, and West Virginia.

WHAT IS HARVESTED AND WHEN: Leaves and roots, in spring and at maturity.

USES: Indians used the roots and leaves to make a tea for treating dizziness and

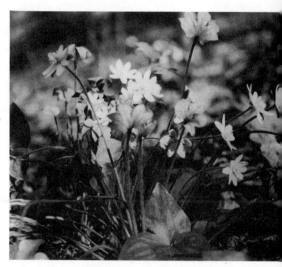

coughs. The roots were chewed to relieve persistent coughs. The plant was used to reduce fever and to treat liver complaints and hemorrhage of the lungs.

COW PARSNIP   135

Heracleum maximum Bartr.

OTHER COMMON NAME: masterwort.

PLANT DESCRIPTION: A perennial growing to 8 feet in height. The plant has a woolly appearance. Its leaves are compound, its flowers white or purple.

WHERE IT GROWS: At all elevations in rich soils. Throughout the United States.

WHAT IS HARVESTED AND WHEN: Roots, of plants more than one year old.

USES: The dried powdered roots have been used on the gums to relieve discomfort from loose teeth, and all over the body to treat fever. Mixed with available fats or oils, the dried powdered roots have been rubbed on affected parts to treat rheumatic pains and heart palpitations. Sometimes the roots have been boiled and the liquid rubbed on for these treatments. The root has been taken internally for colic, gas, diarrhea, indigestion, and asthma.

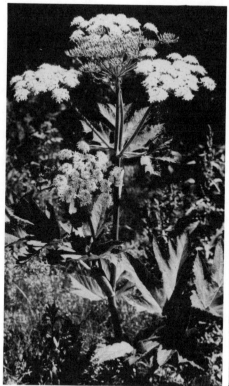

135

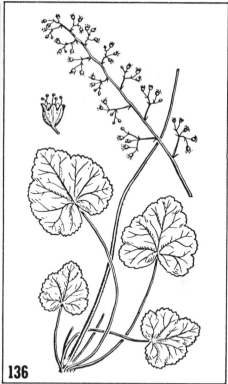

136

ALUMROOT   136

Heuchera americana L.

OTHER COMMON NAMES: American sanicle, cliff-weed, common alumroot, ground maple, rock geranium, split-rock.

PLANT DESCRIPTION: A perennial with a flowering stem, growing to 4 feet in height. The leaves are ½ inch long and toothed. The flowers are red-tinged or greenish, sometimes with purple petals.

WHERE IT GROWS: Shaded woody areas and rock slopes. Connecticut south to Tennessee, Arkansas, and Alabama; west to Michigan, Indiana, Illinois, Missouri, and Oklahoma.

WHAT IS HARVESTED AND WHEN: Roots, of plants more than one year old; leaves, as needed.

USES: A decoction of the root was used in the 1800's as a treatment for sore throat, and by Indians as a poultice on skin lesions and wounds. An infusion of the root was used to treat diarrhea, and a leaf poultice for skin abrasions.

Humulus lupulus L.

The wild form is known as *Humulus lupulus* var. neomexicanus Nels & Cockerell, *Humulus americanus* Nutt., and *Humulus neomexicanus* (Nels. and Cockerell).

OTHER COMMON NAMES: European hop, hop, hopvine, northern vine.

PLANT DESCRIPTION: A twining perennial growing to 20 feet or more. The three-lobed leaves are smooth, 4 to 5 inches long, with stems about 3 inches long. The fruit is membranous and cone-like.

WHERE IT GROWS: Often as a cultivated crop in fields, also in a wide range of habitats, including open fields, roadsides, and abandoned farms. All parts of the United States.

WHAT IS HARVESTED AND WHEN: Fruit (called hops), in the fall.

USES: Both the hops and a powder found in the hops are utilized. Legend has it that King George III of England used a pillow filled with hops to induce sleep. Hot poultices of the hops or powder have been applied to treat painful boils and inflammations. They have also been used to treat fever, intestinal worms, and rheumatism; to increase urine flow; and as a sedative.

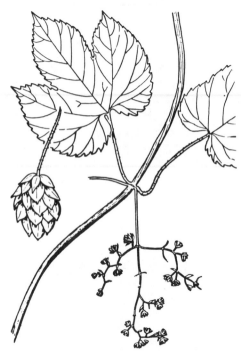

Hydrangea arborescens L.

OTHER COMMON NAMES: sevenbar, wild hydrangea.

PLANT DESCRIPTION: A perennial shrub that grows to 10 feet in height, with stems arising from the base of the plant. It has large, opposite, ovate leaves, and produces white or greenish flowers at the tops of the branches. Many varieties are recognized.

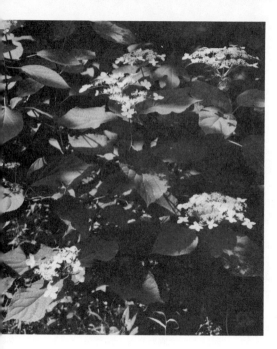

WHERE IT GROWS: Rich woods, calcareous soils, rocky slopes, and banks of streams. New York to Missouri and Oklahoma; south to Georgia, Mississippi, Arkansas, Florida, and Louisiana.

WHAT IS HARVESTED AND WHEN: Roots, in the fall.

USES: Indians made a decoction of the roots and other plant materials and gave it to women who had unusual dreams during their menstrual periods. The roots and rhizomes have been used to increase urine flow and as a tonic and laxative. In colonial times, they were used to treat kidney stones.

GOLDENSEAL   139

Hydrastis canadensis L.

OTHER COMMON NAMES: eyebalm, eyebright, eyeroot, goldenroot, ground raspberry, hydrastis, Indian dye, Indian paint, Indian plant, Indian turmeric, jaundice root, Ohio curcuma, turmeric, wild turmeric, yellow eyewright, yellow painroot, yellow puccoon, yellowwort.

PLANT DESCRIPTION: A perennial that grows to 1 foot in height. It has one stem with two five- to seven-lobed leaves near the top, where a greenish white flower appears. Several single leafstalks, topped with flowers that have no petals, arise from the roots. The fruit looks like a raspberry but is inedible.

WHERE IT GROWS: Rich, shady woods. In the mountains of North Carolina and South Carolina, the Appalachian highlands

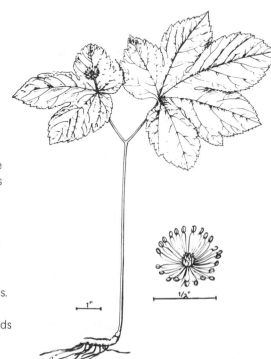

of Kentucky, Tennessee, and West Virginia; Vermont to Minnesota and Nebraska; south to Georgia, Alabama, Arkansas, and Kansas. It has been grown under cultivation in the state of Washington.

WHAT IS HARVESTED AND WHEN: Rootstocks, in the fall; leaves and tops, in late summer or fall after the seeds ripen.

USES: In Appalachia, a root tea is used as a tonic and to improve the appetite. A watery infusion of the roots was used by Indians and pioneers to treat watering eyes. Powdered roots were applied over open cuts and wounds to encourage the formation of scabs. Appalachian Cherokees mixed this same powder with bear grease and rubbed it on the skin as an insect repellent. The pioneers chewed the roots to heal a sore mouth. An infusion of leaves was also used to treat liver and stomach ailments.

AMERICAN HOLLY   140 A

Ilex opaca Ait.

OTHER COMMON NAMES: boxwood, evergreen holly, holly, white holly.

PLANT DESCRIPTION: An evergreen tree growing to 50 feet in height. There are distinct male and female trees, the female bearing bright red berries. The leaves are 2 to 4 inches long, with spiny teeth, green above and yellowish green below.

WHERE IT GROWS: From dry soils on the margins of hardwood forests to areas of rich, moist swamps. Massachusetts, south to Florida and west to Missouri, Oklahoma, and Texas.

WHAT IS HARVESTED AND WHEN: Fruits, when ripe (they remain long on the tree and eventually may shrivel and drop); root bark and bark, in summer and early fall.

USES: In the last century, fresh bark and fruits were gathered before the first frost, chopped to a pulp, mixed with two parts by weight of alcohol, put into a stoppered bottle, and allowed to stand eight days in a dark, cool place, then filtered. This decoction was considered useful as a laxative, and for treating worms, coughs, pleurisy, constipation, fever, gout, rheumatism, and tumors. A decoction of the root bark has been used to treat colds, coughs, and tuberculosis.

YAUPON   140 B

Ilex vomitoria Ait.

OTHER COMMON NAMES: Appalachian tea, Carolina tea, cassena, cassena bush, cassine, cassio-berry bush, deerberry, emetic holly, evergreen cassena, Indian black drink, true cassena, yapon, yopon.

PLANT DESCRIPTION: A much-branched evergreen shrub or small tree growing to a height of 25 feet. The leaves are ½ to 2 inches long, shiny above. The flowers are white, in clusters; the fruits are red or orange, about ¼ inch in diameter.

WHERE IT GROWS: It is common in maritime forests and sometimes found in sandy areas. Virginia to Florida, Alabama, Mississippi, Arkansas, and Texas.

WHAT IS HARVESTED AND WHEN: Leaves, usually in spring.

USES: Indians have made an infusion of the leaves to serve as a laxative. Tribes would visit coastal areas to harvest the leaves for their "black drink" at the end of winter. There have been suggestions that this drink, in addition to serving as a "winter cleaner" and tonic, was slightly narcotic.

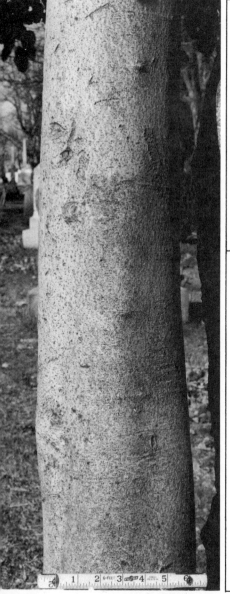

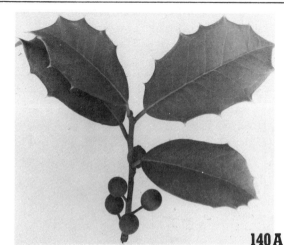

140 A

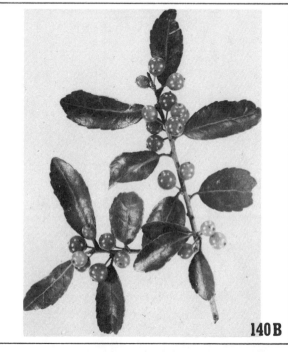

140 B

Ipomoea purpurea (L.) Roth.

PLANT DESCRIPTION: A twining annual with hairy stalks, leaves 3 to 5 inches long, broad at the base and coming to a point. Flowers are blue, violet, or white, 2 to 4 inches across.

WHERE IT GROWS: Fields, roadsides, gardens, fence rows, and waste places. Throughout the United States.

WHAT IS HARVESTED AND WHEN: Roots and stems, as needed; flowers and seeds, in the spring.

USES: At times people have indulged in the dangerous practice of chewing the seeds for hallucinogenic purposes. The flowers, seeds, roots, and stems have been used as a strong laxative.

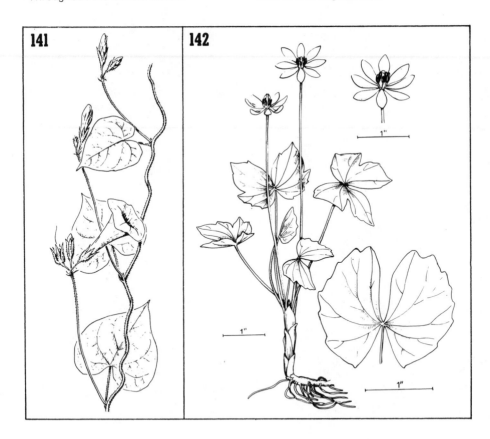

AMERICAN TWINLEAF   142

Jeffersonia diphylla (L.) Pers.

OTHER COMMON NAMES: ground squirrel pea, helmet pod, rheumatism root, twinleaf, yellow root.

PLANT DESCRIPTION: An erect shrub that grows to 2 feet in height. The stalk is topped by two identical, opposite, semicircular leaf segments. The flowers are white, 1 inch across. The fruit is a large capsule.

WHERE IT GROWS: Rich, damp, shaded woods. New York to Wisconsin and Iowa, south to Alabama, including Kentucky, Tennessee, West Virginia, Virginia, and North Carolina.

WHAT IS HARVESTED AND WHEN: Roots, in the fall.

USES: The root is said to induce vomiting in large doses, and to be an effective expectorant in small doses. It has been used as a gargle for sore throat, as a treatment for rheumatism and muscular spasms; to increase urine flow, and to treat syphilis, cramps, ulcers, and mild cases of scarlet fever.

BUTTERNUT   143

Juglans cinerea L.

OTHER NAMES: filnut, lemonnut, oilnut, white walnut.

PLANT DESCRIPTION: A tree that grows to a height of 40 to 60 feet. The bark is light gray, divided into broad, flat ridges, with moderately deep furrows. The leaves are compound, with eleven to seventeen opposite leaflets 2 to 3 inches long, with very short stems. The elliptical, pointed fruit is 1½ inches long, single or in clusters of two to five. The strong-smelling, sticky husk is covered with hairs and contains an edible nut in a hard, thick, deeply furrowed shell.

WHERE IT GROWS: In rich woods and along rivers on well-drained soils. Throughout New England, except Maine; south to New Jersey, Maryland,

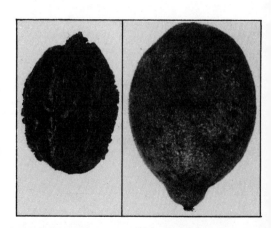

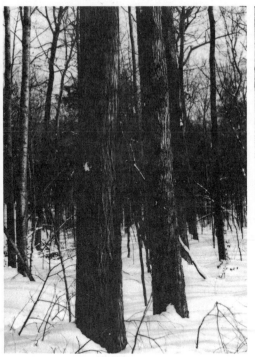

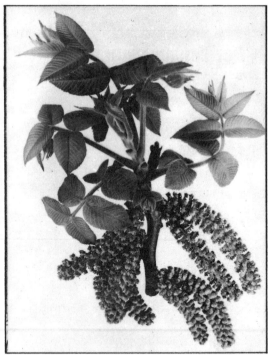

Virginia, North and South Carolina, Georgia, Alabama, Mississippi, and Arkansas; west to Iowa, Minnesota, Wisconsin, and Michigan.

WHAT IS HARVESTED AND WHEN:
Inner bark of roots and trunk and outer bark, usually during the growing season;

fruits, in early fall as they ripen.

USES: The inner bark is considered a cathartic, and in Appalachia a tea is made of it. An oil extracted from the fruit is reportedly useful in treating tapeworms and fungus infections.

BLACK WALNUT   144

Juglans nigra L.

OTHER COMMON NAMES: American walnut, eastern black walnut, walnut.

PLANT DESCRIPTION: A valuable timber tree that often grows to more than 120 feet in height, with almost black bark divided into rough ridges by deep, narrow furrows. The leaflets are alternate, twelve to twenty-three per stem, finely toothed,

and 3 to 3½ inches long. The fruit (nut) occurs singly or in clusters of two or three, and has a thick, fleshy, aromatic husk; it is roundish, about 1½ to 2 inches in diameter, edible, and has a hard, rough, deeply furrowed shell.

WHERE IT GROWS: Rich woods and limestone soils. Throughout the Eastern

United States as far north as southern Michigan, Minnesota, and Wisconsin, southern New York, Vermont, Massachusetts, and Connecticut, south to Florida, Mississippi, and Louisiana; west to Arkansas, Oklahoma, Texas, Kansas, and South Dakota.

WHAT IS HARVESTED AND WHEN:
Bark, in spring or fall; fruit, in late summer or early fall; leaves, as required.

USES: The inner bark of the tree is a mild laxative, and was used commonly during the American Revolution. The peel of the fruit is reputed to be useful for treating intestinal worms, ulcers, and syphilis. The juice of the fruit is considered useful for treating tapeworms, as a laxative, and as a gargle in treating diphtheria. A leaf infusion is used against bedbugs.

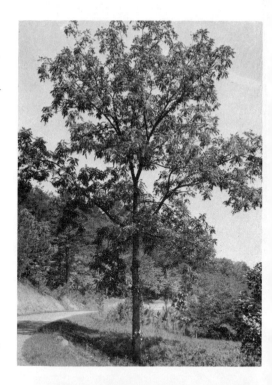

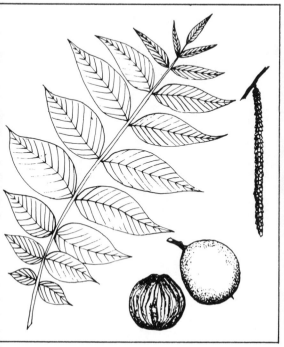

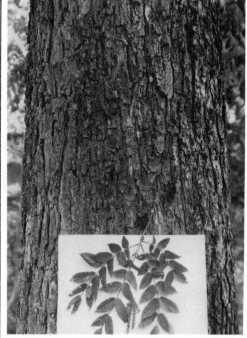

COMMON JUNIPER   145

Juniperus communis L.

OTHER COMMON NAMES: dwarf juniper, gorst, ground juniper, hackmatack, horse savin, juniper, juniper bush, prostrate juniper, scent cedar, scrub juniper.

PLANT DESCRIPTION: A small-evergreen shrub or tree 12 to 30 feet in height, low and spreading or upright. The bark of the trunk is reddish brown and tends to shred. The needles are straight, sharp-pointed, ridged, and nearly at right angles to the branchlets. The fruit is dark purple, round, about ¼ inch in diameter, fleshy and berry-like.

WHERE IT GROWS: Dry, sterile hills, dry woods, old fields, dried bogs,

coastal dunes, and exposed rocky areas. The tree is widely distributed from New Mexico to the Dakotas and eastward.

WHAT IS HARVESTED AND WHEN: Fruits, in fall and winter; foliage, as needed; wood, after trees are cut down.

USES: The fruit is used to increase urination, induce menstruation, relieve gas and colic, and treat kidney complaints, snakebite, and intestinal worms. Indians used a poultice made of needles and twigs to treat wounds. The wood yields cedar oil, formerly used to treat chronic disorders of the genitourinary tract.

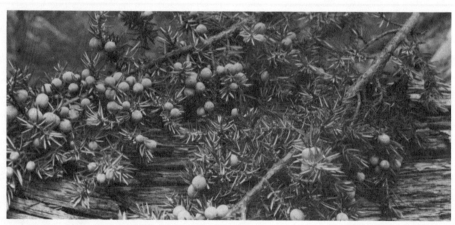

EASTERN REDCEDAR   146

Juniperus virginiana L.

OTHER COMMON NAMES: Carolina cedar, cedar, cedar apple, evergreen, juniper, pencil cedar, red cedar, red juniper, red savin, savin, Virginia cedar.

PLANT DESCRIPTION: This evergreen tree can grow to over 100 feet in height on good sites, but may barely reach 20 feet on dry sites in the prairie region. The leafy twigs are rounded, four-angled, and slender. There are two kinds of leaves: the younger ones are needle-shaped, 1/8 to 1/4 inch long, and occur opposite each other; the adult needles are scalelike and 1/2 inch long. The highly aromatic, dark blue cone, fleshy and berry-like, has one or two small seeds.

WHERE IT GROWS: Pasture land, dry, open woods, rocky slopes, and barren areas. Throughout the eastern United States; south to Kentucky, Tennessee, coastal Georgia, Alabama, and Mississippi; west to Michigan, the Dakotas, Kansas, Texas, and New Mexico.

WHAT IS HARVESTED AND WHEN: Leaves and twigs, during the growing season; fruits and nuts, in late summer and early fall.

USES: In Appalachia, a mixture of seeds, leaves, and twigs is boiled and the steam inhaled as a treatment for bronchitis. Indians used a decoction of boiled fruit and leaves for coughs, a warm poultice of boiled sprigs and leaves for rheumatism, and a tea of boiled leaves for convalescence and weakness. The decoction has been used as a stimulant, to treat menstrual delay and to induce perspiration. Use of the oil to induce abortion has proved fatal. Spanish-speaking New Mexicans have used a boiled mixture of bark and water to treat skin rash.

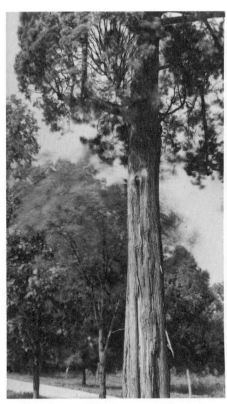
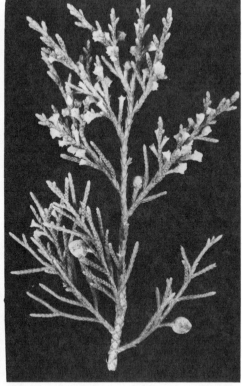

Kallstroemia grandiflora Torr.

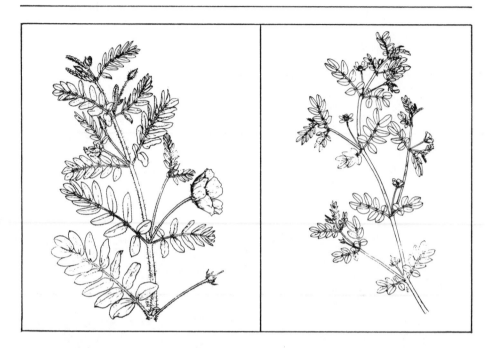

PLANT DESCRIPTION: A prostrate annual with opposite leaves and small yellow flowers. Sepals are present under the fruit, which is 1½ inches long, splitting into ten one-seeded parts.

WHERE IT GROWS: Dry plains. New Mexico and Texas.

WHAT IS HARVESTED AND WHEN: Roots, in the fall; leaves, as needed.

USES: Indians chewed the leaves for toothache, and applied a poultice of them to skin sores and bruises. The powdered root in warm water was used as a wash for sore eyes. A tea made of the root was used for stomachache, diarrhea, and fever. In Central America, young plants are eaten as a vegatable.

Kalmia latifolia L.

OTHER COMMON NAMES: big-leaved ivy, calico-bush, calico flower, calico-tree, dog bush, dogwood, ivy, kalmia, laurel, mountain ivy, poison ivy, poison laurel, sheep laurel, small laurel, spoon wood, wood laurel.

PLANT DESCRIPTION: An evergreen shrub usually to 10 or 15 feet in height, but sometimes as high as 30 feet. It has dense, round-topped, waxy leaves, dark green above and yellowish green below, 2 to 5 inches long. The flowers, in flat-topped clusters, are rose-colored to white, with purple markings, ¾ inch across.

WHERE IT GROWS: Rocky or gravel-ly woods, clearings, swamps, and mountainsides. New England, New York, Ohio, and Indiana, south to Florida and Louisiana.

WHAT IS HARVESTED AND WHEN: Leaves, when plant is in bloom.

USES: The powdered leaves mixed with lard have been used to treat skin rashes and infections. It was believed at one time that Indians drank a decoction of the leaves as a suicide potion. In the 1800's, a tincture of the leaves was prescribed for syphilis, diarrhea, skin eruptions, and eye diseases.

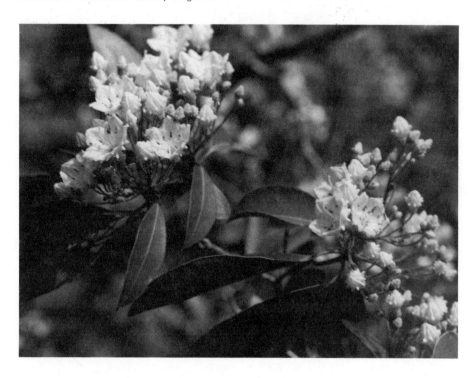

Lactuca scariola L.

OTHER COMMON NAMES: compass plant, wild lettuce, wild opium.

PLANT DESCRIPTION: An annual or perennial with a single stalk, usually growing to 2 feet in height. The flowers are yellow, turning purple or blue when dried. The leaves are cleft, with deep lobes.

Leaves and plant, in summer or fall; milky juice of the stem, in summer.

USES: The whole plant has been used to increase urine flow and to soothe sore and chapped skin. Indians made a tea from the leaves and used it to hasten the milk flow of new mothers. Early settlers used

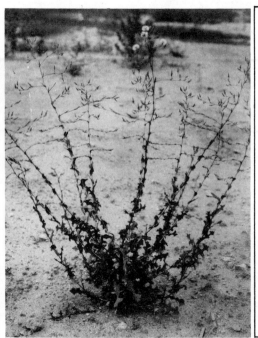
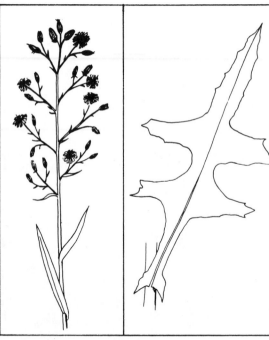

WHERE IT GROWS: Roadsides, dry soils and gardens, and waste areas. Throughout the United States.

WHAT IS HARVESTED AND WHEN:

the juice as a sedative and nerve tonic. At one time, the milky sap was thought to be useful as a substitute for opium, but this idea never gained ground.

AMERICAN LARIX   150

Larix laricina (DuRoi) K. Koch.

OTHER COMMON NAMES: black larch, black larix, eastern larch, hackmatack, hacmack, juniper, larch, red larch, tamarack.

PLANT DESCRIPTION: An evergreen tree that grows to 60 feet in height, with horizontal branches and reddish bark. The needles are bluish green, 1½ inches long. The cones are rounded, ¾ inch long.

WHERE IT GROWS: Swamps, bogs, and damp, forested areas. New England, New Jersey, Pennsylvania, and West Virginia; west to Ohio, Indiana, Illinois, Michigan, and Minnesota.

WHAT IS HARVESTED AND WHEN: Bark, as needed; gum, as available.

USES: The gum that exudes from the bark has been chewed to relieve indigestion. The bark has been used as a laxative and tonic and to treat rheumatism and jaundice. A poultice of the bark has been used for bruises and wounds.

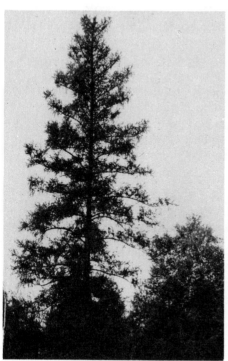
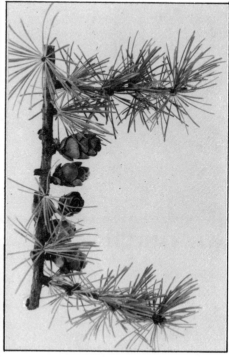

MOTHERWORT 151

Leonurus cardiaca L.

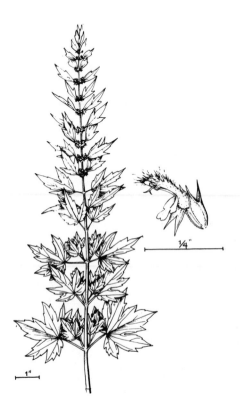

OTHER COMMON NAMES: common motherwort, lion's ear, lion's tail, lion's tart, throwwort.

PLANT DESCRIPTION: A perennial that grows to 5 or 6 feet in height. The leaves are up to 5 inches in length, lobed and dentate. The flowers are white to pink and very fuzzy.

WHERE IT GROWS: Pastures, waste places, and roadsides. Northeastern states; west to Montana and Texas; south to North Carolina and Tennessee.

WHAT IS HARVESTED AND WHEN: Above-ground parts, at flowering time.

USES: In Russia, this plant was considered effective for treating rabies. It has been used in the United States as a stimulant and tonic, and to increase urine flow. Europeans have used it for asthma and heart palpitations. It is usually taken as an infusion.

COMMON SPICEBUSH 152

Lindera benzoin (L.) Blume

OTHER COMMON NAMES: allspice bush, Benjamin bush, feverbush, spiceberry, spicebush, wild allspice.

PLANT DESCRIPTION: A deciduous shrub that grows to 15 feet in height. The aromatic leaves are 3 to 5 inches long

and alternate. The greenish yellow flowers occur in dense clusters, producing long, bright red berries.

WHERE IT GROWS: Damp woods and stream banks. New England south to Kentucky, Tennessee, and North Carolina;

west to Missouri and Kansas; north to Michigan and Illinois.

WHAT IS HARVESTED AND WHEN:
Barks and twigs, as needed; fruit, when ripe.

USES: A decoction of the bark, twigs, or fruit was used to stimulate blood circulation, increase perspiration, and treat for intestinal worms, dysentery, coughs, and colds. In the Revolutionary period, the fruit was used as a substitute for allspice. In the South, during the Civil War, the leaves were used as a substitute for tea.

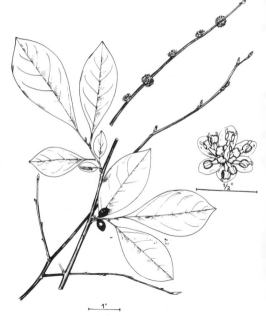

SWEETGUM   153

Liquidambar styraciflua L.

OTHER COMMON NAMES: alligator tree, American mahogany, American storax, American sweetgum, bilsted, gum, gumwood, gum-tree, hazelwood, incense tree, liquidambar, liquid storax, opossum-tree, redgum, sap, sapgum, satin walnut, satin wood, star leaf gum, star-leaved gum, storax tree, styrax, sycamore gum, white gum.

PLANT DESCRIPTION: A tree that grows to 125 feet in height. The leaves

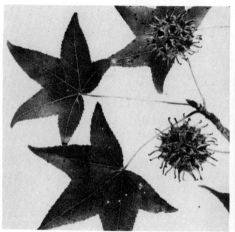

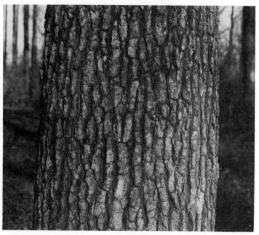

are star-shaped, with five pointed lobes. The fruit is contained in woody, spiky, globular capsules. The seeds are winged.

WHERE IT GROWS: River bottoms, moist and alluvial areas, and swampy woods. Connecticut to Florida, to Texas, Missouri, Arkansas, and Oklahoma, and north to Illinois.

WHAT IS HARVESTED AND WHEN: Gum from the tree trunk, as it appears; bark, in spring or fall; leaves and twigs, during the growing season.

USES: In Appalachia, water- or whiskey-soaked twigs are chewed to clean the teeth. Indians used the resin to treat fevers and wounds. The gum was used by early settlers to treat herpes and skin inflammations. It has also been applied to the cheek to ease toothache. The bark and leaves, boiled in milk or water, have been used to treat diarrhea and dysentery. The boiled leaves have been applied to cuts and used for treating sore feet. The drug storax, an expectorant and a weak antiseptic used for treating scabies, comes from this tree.

YELLOW-POPLAR   154

Liriodendron tulipifera L.

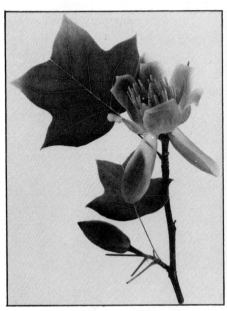 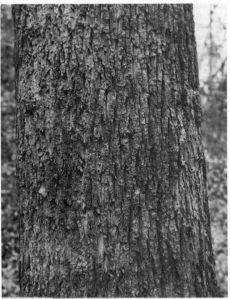

OTHER COMMON NAMES: basswood, blue poplar, canary yellow-wood, canoewood, cucumbertree, hickory poplar, old wife's shirt tree, poplar, popple, saddleleaf, saddletree, sap poplar, soft yellow poplar, tulippoplar, tulip tree, tulip wood, white poplar, whitewood.

PLANT DESCRIPTION: A tree that may grow to over 100 feet in height. Its flowers are greenish yellow, orange within, 2 inches long. The fruit is brown, conelike, and up to 3 inches long.

WHERE IT GROWS: Deep, organic soils, near streams, on mountain slopes. New England to Michigan, south to Florida and Louisiana.

WHAT IS HARVESTED AND WHEN: Buds, in early spring; bark from roots, trunk, leaves, and branches, during the growing season.

USES: An ointment made of the buds crushed in grease was used to treat scalds, burns, and inflammations. The crushed leaves were used as a poultice to treat headaches. A decoction of the root bark was applied warm to an infected tooth for relief of pain. It has also been used in treating rheumatism, malaria, and hysteria. The inner bark was once considered a stimulant.

INDIAN TOBACCO   155

Lobelia inflata L.

OTHER COMMON NAMES: asthma weed, bladder pod, bladder-podded lobelia, emetic herb, emetic weed, eyebright, field lobelia, gagroot, Indian tobacco lobelia, lobelia, obelia, pukeweed, tobacco lobelia, vomitwort, wild tobacco.

PLANT DESCRIPTION: A branching annual that grows to 3 feet in height, with leaves 1 to 3 inches long and small

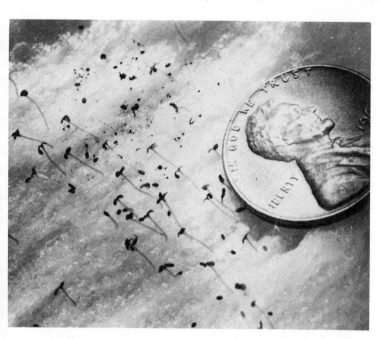
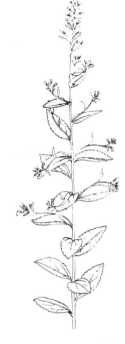

violet to pinkish white flowers, borne in the axils of the leaves. The bottoms of the flowers inflate to form a seed capsule with many very tiny, brown, shiny seeds.

WHERE IT GROWS: In dry, open fields, woods, roadsides, and partial shade. New England into Appalachia; south to Geogia, Mississippi, and Alabama; west to Kansas and Arkansas; north to Minnesota.

WHAT IS HARVESTED AND WHEN: Entire plant, at full bloom or when seed capsules are present.

USES: An alkaloid, lobeline, is extracted from the plant and used in various anti-smoking preparations. Indians used the powdered leaves to treat.dysentery. The plant has been used to treat whooping cough, asthma, epilepsy, pneumonia, hysteria, and convulsions.

GREAT LOBELIA 156

Lobelia siphilitica L.

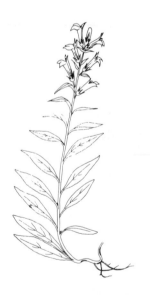

OTHER COMMON NAMES: big blue lobelia, blue cardinal flower, blue cardinal lobelia, blue lobelia cardinal, cardinal, highbelia, Louisiana lobelia.

PLANT DESCRIPTION: An unbranched perennial growing to 3 feet in height. The leaves are 5 to 6 inches long; the flowers deep lilac to purple, ¾ inch long, in long spikes.

WHERE IT GROWS: Rich, low woods, stream banks, wet places, and dense forests. New England, south to Florida, Mississippi, Missouri, and Kansas.

WHAT IS HARVESTED AND WHEN: Above-ground plants, at full bloom; roots, as needed.

USES: Indians used the plant and roots to treat syphilis and gonorrhea, in combination with mayapple (*Podophyllum peltatum*) roots. The plant was also used to clear the chest of phlegm, to induce vomiting, to treat dysentery, and to increase urine flow.

Lycopodium clavatum L.

OTHER COMMON NAMES: clubfoot moss, club moss, foxtail, ground pine, hog's bed, lamb's tail, running club moss, running pine, snake moss, stag's horn, vegetable sulfur moss, wolf's claw.

PLANT DESCRIPTION: A very low-growing evergreen perennial resembling moss. The leaves often have a bristle at the apex. The plant has no flowers but produces yellow spores.

WHERE IT GROWS: The several varieties are found in all sorts of localities, from barren hills to woods. The plant has a wide range over all the states, including Alaska.

WHAT IS HARVESTED AND WHEN: Spores, as available.

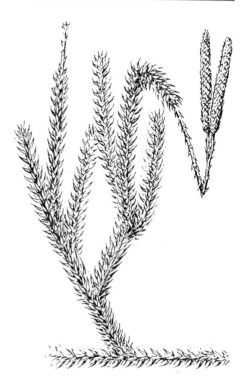

USES: The spores have been used in decoctions to increase urine flow, to treat severe diarrhea, and to increase the appetite in certain nervous troubles, and have been considered an aphrodisiac. As a dusting powder, the spores have been used on babies' skin to prevent chafing.

Lycopus virginicus L.

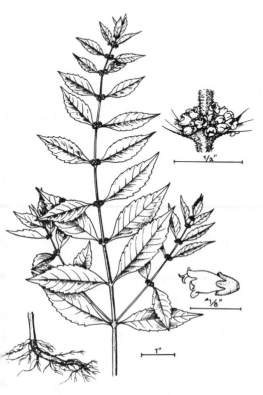

gypsywort, horehound, Paul's betony, purple archangel, sweet bugleweed, water bugle, water horehound, wolf foot, wood betony.

PLANT DESCRIPTION: A shrub with dark green, purplish-tinged leaves, which are coarsely toothed and narrow at each end. The flowers are tubular, borne in the leaf axils, and the fruits are small nutlets.

WHERE IT GROWS: Rich, moist forests, swampy areas, and fields. Maine, New Hampshire, Vermont, New York, Ohio, Indiana, Wisconsin, Minnesota, and Nebraska, south to Texas, east to Georgia.

WHAT IS HARVESTED AND WHEN: Entire plant at full bloom, in summer or fall.

USES: The plant has been reported to be a sedative and has been used to treat diabetes, diarrhea, tuberculosis, and pulmonary hemorrhaging.

OTHER COMMON NAMES: bugleweed, buglewort, carpenter's herb, gypsyweed,

Maclura pomifera (Raf.) Schneid.

OTHER COMMON NAMES: bodeck, bodoch, bois d'arc, bow-wood osage appletree, hedge, hedge apple, hedge-osage, hedge-plant osage, horse apple, mockorange, orange-like maclura, osage apple, wild orange.

PLANT DESCRIPTION: A tree or shrub growing to 30 feet in height. The leaves are 2 to 5 inches long, with spines in the leaf axils. The fruit is 4 to 5 inches in diameter and resembles a large orange, greenish to yellow in color.

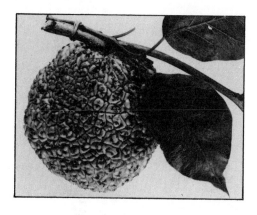

WHERE IT GROWS: Rich bottomlands and moist areas, fence rows, and roadsides. Northeast and Midwest, to Texas and Arkansas.

WHAT IS HARVESTED AND WHEN: Roots, as needed.

USES: The boiled root yielded a decoction once used to bathe irritated eyes.

SWEETBAY MAGNOLIA   160

Magnolia virginiana L.

OTHER COMMON NAMES: bay, beavertree, bog beaver, brewster, castor wood, Indian bark, laurel-magnolia, magnolia, small magnolia, swampbay, swamp laurel, swamp sassafras, sweet-bay, white bay, white laurel.

PLANT DESCRIPTION: A tree growing to 60 feet in height, evergreen in the South and deciduous in the northern states. The leaves are 3 to 6 inches long, white or gray below, green above. The flowers are white, round, fragrant, 2 to

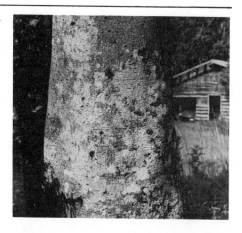

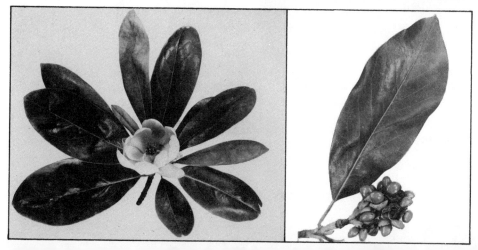

3 inches across. The fruit is red and 1 to 2 inches long.

WHERE IT GROWS: Woods and margins of swamps. Massachusetts to Florida and the Texas coast.

WHAT IS HARVESTED AND WHEN: Cones and seeds, in late summer and fall as they ripen; leaves, as they mature; bark, as needed; root bark, in spring and fall.

USES: Indians drank a warm infusion of the bark, cones, and seeds for rheumatism. In colonial times, the root bark was used in place of quinine bark to treat malaria. A drink made of an infusion of bark and brandy was used to treat lung and chest diseases, dysentery, and fever. A tea made of young branches boiled in water was a treatment for colds. The bark and fruit are aromatic and have been used as a tonic. A tincture of the fresh leaves has been used to treat rheumatism and gout, and as a laxative.

LITTLE MALLOW   161

Malva parviflora L.

OTHER COMMON NAMES: cheeseweed, malva del campo, malva mexicana.

PLANT DESCRIPTION: An annual or biennial growing to 4 feet in height. The small, pinkish flowers appear in clusters in leaf axils.

WHERE IT GROWS: Orchards and waste places. New England to New Jersey; North Dakota to the Pacific Northwest; south to Texas, New Mexico, and Missouri.

WHAT IS HARVESTED AND WHEN: Leaves, as they mature; whole plant, when in bloom.

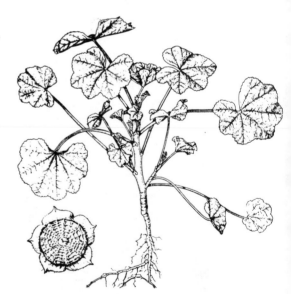

USES: The bruised leaves have been rubbed on the skin to treat skin irritations. A strained tea of the boiled leaves has been administered after childbirth to clean out the mother's system. As a headache remedy, the leaves or the whole plant have been mashed and placed on the forehead. Powdered leaves have been blown into the throat to treat swollen glands. The leaves have been used to induce perspiration and menstrual flow, reduce fever, and treat pneumonia.

WHITE HOREHOUND   162

Marrubium vulgare L.

OTHER COMMON NAMES: common hoarhound, common horehound, hoarhound, horehound, houndsbane, marrhue, marrub, marrubium, marvel, white hoarhound.

PLANT DESCRIPTION: A shrub that grows to 3 feet in height, with ovate-round, fuzzy leaves, whitish above and gray below. The foliage is aromatic when crushed.

WHERE IT GROWS: Pastures, old fields, and waste places. In almost all of the United States, except the more arid parts of the Southwest.

WHAT IS HARVESTED AND WHEN: Leaves and small stems, in May before blooming; bark, as needed.

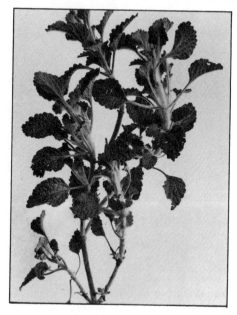

USES: In Appalachia, the leaves are combined with honey to make a syrup for treating coughs. The dried bark is used to make a tea to treat colds and debility. A warm infusion has been used as a tonic. The plant is considered to be a mild laxative and has been used to treat asthma, diarrhea, menstrual irregularity, and kidney ailments.

CAJEPUT TREE   163

Melaleuca leucadendra L.

OTHER COMMON NAMES: punk tree, swamp tea tree.

PLANT DESCRIPTION: An evergreen tree growing to 50 feet in height, with white bark. The leaves are 3 to 8 inches long, deep green, and aromatic. The flowers are whitish to pink and purple, lacking stalks.

WHERE IT GROWS: Introduced from Burma and Malaya, this plant is found in Florida.

WHAT IS HARVESTED AND WHEN: Young twigs and leaves, as needed.

USES: Cajeput oil is distilled from the fresh twigs and leaves and is used externally to treat scabies and other parasitic skin diseases. The oil is put into a tooth cavity to relieve toothache. It has been used as an insect repellent, to cure headache and earache, to expel worms from the intestines, and to clear phlegm from the chest area. In India, a tea is made from the leaves.

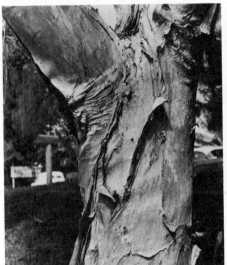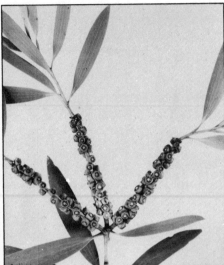

COMMON MOONSEED   164

Menispermum canadense L.

OTHER COMMON NAMES: Canada moonseed, maple vine, moonseed, Texas sarsaparilla, vine maple, yellow parilla, yellow sarsaparilla.

PLANT DESCRIPTION: A woody climbing perennial vine with wide leaves, lobed around the outside margins. The white to green flowers, in clusters, give rise to clusters of small black berries.

WHERE IT GROWS: Rich alluvial soils, stream beds, woodlands, fence rows, and ravines. New England and the northeastern states to Georgia and Oklahoma.

WHAT IS HARVESTED AND WHEN: Rhizomes and roots, in the fall.

USES: A tincture of the fresh roots has been used as a laxative and for treatment

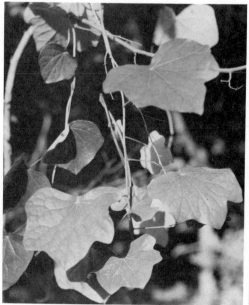
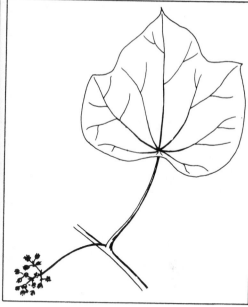

of syphilis, rheumatism, gout, and skin infections. The roots have been used as a substitute for sarsaparilla and are said to have tonic properties and to increase urine flow. As a drink, it was used in pioneer times to treat weakness resulting from prolonged illness.

PEPPERMINT   165

Mentha piperita L.

OTHER COMMON NAMES: brandy mint, lamb mint, lammint.

PLANT DESCRIPTION: A perennial that grows to 3½ feet in height. It has a strong minty flavor and dark green, toothed leaves. The purplish flowers are produced in spikelike groups along the stem in leaf axils and at the top.

WHERE IT GROWS: Shady, damp areas, brook banks, marshes, ditches, old orchards, wet meadows, and stream banks. All parts of the United States (except the Rocky Mountain states, Arizona), New Mexico, Nevada, and the plains states .

WHAT IS HARVESTED AND WHEN: Fresh flowering tops, at full bloom.

USES: Peppermint oil is a product of this plant, which was cultivated first in England in the 1700's and in the United States somewhat later. In Appalachia, the plant has been made into a tea used to treat indigestion and colic. Peppermint has been considered a stimulant and used for all sorts of intestinal ailments. The oil is rubbed on sore spots and strained muscles, and is used for treating muscular aches and rheumatism.

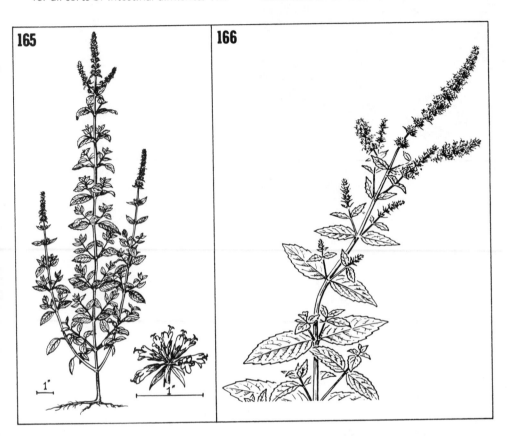

SPEARMINT 166

Mentha spicata L.

OTHER COMMON NAMES: brown mint, common mint, garden mint, lady's mint, our lady's mint, sage of Bethlehem, Scotch mint, Scotch spearmint, yerba-buena.

PLANT DESCRIPTION: A perennial that grows to 3 feet in height, resembling other mints but differing in taste and smell. The flowers are white or pink, borne in long spikes both in upper leaf axils and at the top of the plant.

WHERE IT GROWS: Damp places, throughout the United States.

WHAT IS HARVESTED AND WHEN: Above-ground parts, when plant is in bloom.

USES: The Indians used a spearmint tea for indigestion, diarrhea, and neuralgia, and also washed sores with it. This practice was passed on to the Spanish-speaking New Mexicans, who call spearmint *yerba buena*—"the good plant." These descendants of the Spanish colonizers make a tea of the leaves, add cinnamon, and give it to expectant mothers. The Maya believed this treatment would hasten childbirth. The dried tops were also used as a stimulant and to prevent vomiting.

BUCKBEAN   167

Menyanthes trifoliata L.

OTHER COMMON NAMES: Bean trefoil, bitter trefoil, bogbean, bog myrtle, brook bean, marsh clover, marsh trefoil.

PLANT DESCRIPTION: A smooth, perennial marsh plant with a thick rootstock bearing leaves deeply three-lobed. The flowers are white or reddish, with long stalks.

WHERE IT GROWS: Moist woods, marshes and swamps, pond shores. New England to the Appalachians and Virginia, west to Wyoming and Nebraska.

WHAT IS HARVESTED AND WHEN: Entire plant, at full bloom.

USES: An infusion of the plant has been drunk to treat gout, constipation, and rheumatism and to stimulate the appetite. The plant has been used as a treatment for skin eruptions, worms, scurvy, indigestion, and jaundice.

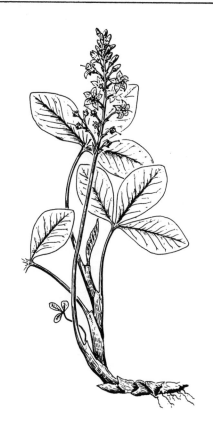

COLORADO FOUR-O'CLOCK   168

Mirabilis multiflora (Torr.) Gray

OTHER COMMON NAME: wild four-o'clock.

PLANT DESCRIPTION: A much-branched perennial growing to a height of 4 feet. The flowers are purplish red to purple, 2 inches long, in groups of as many as six.

WHERE IT GROWS: Partly shaded sites in foothills and valleys between elevations of 4,000 and 9,000 feet. California, Utah, Arizona, New Mexico, and Texas.

WHAT IS HARVESTED AND WHEN: Roots, as needed.

USES: The root has been used as a vision-inducer by western Indians, and the powdered root has been taken to treat stomachache.

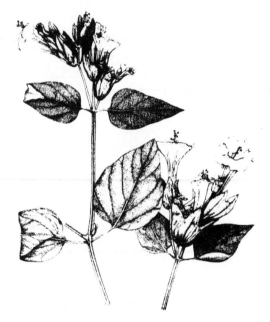

PARTRIDGE BERRY   169

Mitchella repens L.

OTHER COMMON NAMES: checkerberry, creepchequer berry, creeping chequer berry, hive vine, odor berry, one berry, running box, squawberry, squaw vine, twinberry, two-eyed berry, two-eyed chequer berry, winter clover.

PLANT DESCRIPTION: A low-growing perennial vine with roundish evergreen leaves that are shiny above. It produces scented white flowers, tinged with purple, and scarlet berries.

WHERE IT GROWS: Shaded woods, in both moist and dry areas. New England to Minnesota, south to Texas and Florida.

WHAT IS HARVESTED AND WHEN: Entire plant, with fruit, in the fall.

USES: A tea made of the plant has been used for insomnia and excessive water retention, to aid in childbirth, and to alleviate diarrhea.

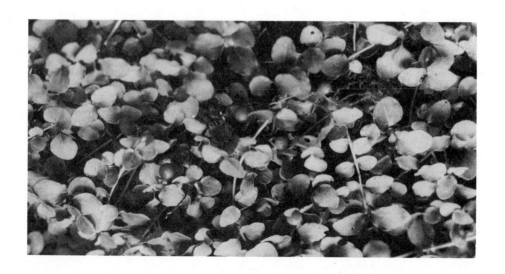

WILD BERGAMOT 170

Monarda fistulosa L.

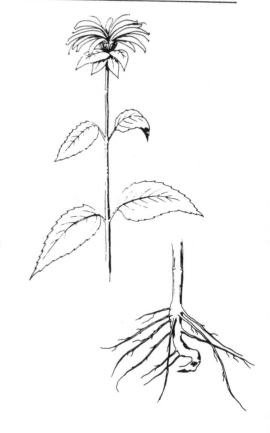

OTHER COMMON NAMES: bee balm, horse mint, long flowered horsemint, oregano, oregano de la Sierra, Oswego tea, purple bergamot.

PLANT DESCRIPTION: An aromatic erect herb, soft and fuzzy, growing to 4 feet in height. The leaves are gray-green and narrow, the upper ones sometimes pink-tinged. The flowers are borne in dense clusters, white to purplish, 1 inch long.

WHERE IT GROWS: Upland woods, thickets, and prairies. New England south to Georgia and Louisiana, west to Texas and Arizona.

WHAT IS HARVESTED AND WHEN: Roots, in spring or fall; leaves, when fully matured; entire above-ground parts, at full bloom or after.

USES: Indians made a decoction of the leaves and treated chills by bathing the patient with it; the dried herb was boiled and the vapors were inhaled for bronchial ailments; a decoction of the root was drunk for stomach disorders; and a tea of leaves and flowers was used for bronchial problems. The pioneers made a lotion of boiled leaves for treating pimples and skin eruptions. A plant infusion has been used to reduce fever and treat headaches, colds, and sore throats. Some Indians in New Mexico dry and pulverize the plant and rub it on the forehead to relieve headache. Also in New Mexico, it is used as a meat flavoring and with beans.

INDIAN-PIPE 171

Monotropa uniflora L.

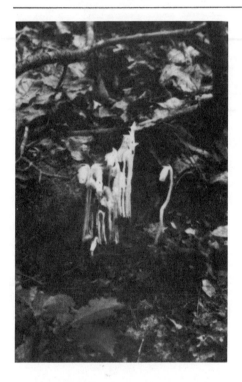

OTHER COMMON NAMES: convulsion-root, corpse plant, fits-root, ghost-flower, pipe plant.

PLANT DESCRIPTION: A succulent, waxy, white plant growing to 1 foot in height. Several stems arise together, often parasitic. The leaves are smooth-edged and tapered. The flowers are single, at the top of the stem, bell-shaped, and up to 1 inch in length. The fruit is a capsule.

WHERE IT GROWS: On woodland humus, decaying organic matter, and the roots of trees. Throughout the United States.

WHAT IS HARVESTED AND WHEN: Roots, as the plants appear; plants, as needed.

USES: The dried powdered root was given to children for epilepsy and convulsions. Indians mixed the juice of the pulverized plant with water and used it as an eye lotion. At one time the dried plant was used in place of opium to relieve pain and induce sleep. Settlers used the fresh juice for a wide range of eye ailments.

Morus alba L.

OTHER COMMON NAMES: Chinese mulberry, silkworm tree, white morus.

PLANT DESCRIPTION: A tree grow-ing to 50 feet in height, with a thick trunk sometimes as much as 2 feet in diameter. The leaves are 3 to 6 inches long, pale green, and irregularly toothed. The fruits are variable in size and color, from 1 to 2 inches long, white to purple, and sweet to the taste.

WHERE IT GROWS: Open areas in woods, meadows, roadsides, old fields. New York south to the Carolinas and to Missouri, Illinois, Indiana, and elsewhere.

WHAT IS HARVESTED AND WHEN: Fruits, when ripe; roots, as needed.

USES: A drink from the fruit has been used to treat high fever, and as a mild lax-ative. The root has been used to make a tea for treating diarrhea.

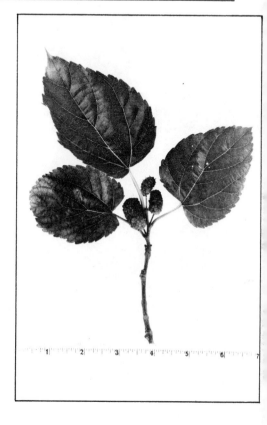

Morus nigra L.

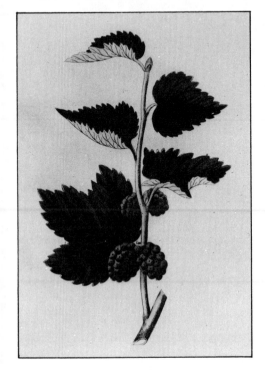

OTHER COMMON NAMES: cel tree, mulberry.

PLANT DESCRIPTION: A small tree growing to 30 feet in height. The leaves, 2 to 8 inches long, are thick, dark dull green, with toothed margins. The fruits are 1 inch long, black or purple.

WHERE IT GROWS: A windbreak or yard tree. Southern United States and California; in protected spots in the Northeast.

WHAT IS HARVESTED AND WHEN: Fruits, when ripe; bark, as needed.

USES: The fruit has been used in drinks prescribed to reduce high fever, and also has been made into a cough syrup. The bark has been used to expel intestinal worms.

RED MULBERRY   174

Morus rubra L.

OTHER COMMON NAMES: black mulberry, bulberry, murier sauvage, Virginia mulberry, Virginia mulberry tree.

PLANT DESCRIPTION: A tree growing to 60 feet in height, with a broad, rounded top. The leaves are 3 to 6 inches long, rough above, fuzzy beneath. The fruits are dark purple to red, up to 1¼ inches in length.

WHERE IT GROWS: Rich cover and edges of woods. New England west to Michigan, South Dakota, and Texas, south to Florida.

WHAT IS HARVESTED AND WHEN: Fruits, in late summer; bark, as needed; sap, during growing season.

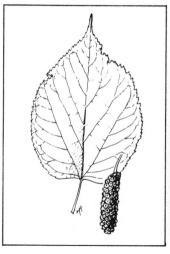
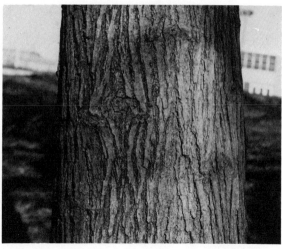

USES: Like other mulberries, the fruit is used to make a cooling drink for fever, as well as for a mild laxative. The outer bark has been used to treat intestinal worms. The inner bark, scraped and boiled as a tea, has been used for a children's laxative. Some Indians used the sap to treat ringworm.

SOUTHERN WAX MYRTLE 175

Myrica cerifera L.

OTHER COMMON NAMES: American vegetable tallow, American vegetable wax, bayberry, bayberry tallow, bayberry waxtree, bearing myrica, candleberry, candleberry myrtle, cirier, myrtle, myrtle tree, puckerbush, southern bayberry, tallow bayberry, tallow shrub, waxberry, wax myrtle.

PLANT DESCRIPTION: A perennial shrub that grows to 30 feet in height, with waxy branchlets. The narrow evergreen leaves taper at both ends. The flowers are borne in catkins. The fruits are grayish berries.

WHERE IT GROWS: Coastal areas, open fields, banks of streams, pine barrens, and low areas. Coastal region from New Jersey, Delaware, and Maryland to Florida, Alabama, Mississippi, and Arkansas.

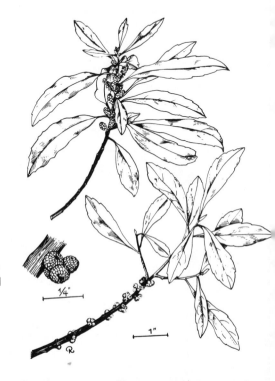

¼"

1"

WHAT IS HARVESTED AND WHEN:
Root bark, in the fall (by gently heating the roots and stripping the bark); leaves, as needed; fruits, in the fall and well into the winter.

USES: Leaves and stems are boiled in water and used to treat fever. A decoction of boiled leaves is used to eliminate intestinal worms. A decoction made from root bark has been used to treat uterine hemorrhage, jaundice, dysentery, cankers of the mouth and throat, and spongy gums. The leaves have provided vitamin C for curing scurvy. The fruit is the main source of the bayberry wax used in candle-making.

WATERCRESS 176

Nasturtium officinale R. Br.

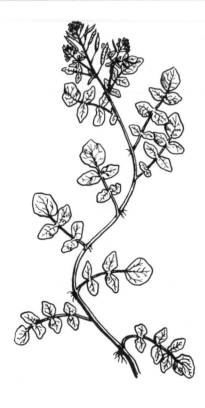

OTHER COMMON NAMES: nasturtium, true watercress.

PLANT DESCRIPTION: A succulent aquatic perennial. Its leaves are light green, alternate, and divided; its stems are thick and hollow.

WHERE IT GROWS: In thick beds in the cold, flowing water of ditches, slow streams, brooks, and ponds. Throughout the United States.

WHAT IS HARVESTED AND WHEN:
Entire plant, when available.

USES: The plant is eaten fresh as a salad and is a fine source of vitamins A and C. Spanish-speaking New Mexicans eat it as a treatment for kidney and heart trouble, and crush it in cold water as a remedy for tuberculosis. The fresh plant has also been used to treat constipation, although pregnant women have been warned not to eat it because it may cause abortion. A cough remedy is made by soaking the cut-up leaves in honey overnight. In Africa, it is believed to cause temporary sterility but has been used as an aphrodisiac and to treat head colds and asthma.

Nepeta cataria L.

OTHER COMMON NAMES: catmint, catnep, catrup, catwort, field balm, nip.

PLANT DESCRIPTION: An erect perennial that grows to 3 feet in height. The stem is downy and whitish, the leaves heart-shaped, opposite, coarsely dentate, 2 to 3 inches long. The flowers are tubular, ¼ to ½ inch long, whitish with purplish markings, occurring in compact spikes.

WHERE IT GROWS: Fence rows, roadsides, waste places, and stream banks. It grows wild in Virginia, Tennessee, West Virginia, Georgia, New England, Illinois, Indiana, Ohio, New Mexico, Colorado, Arizona, Utah, and California. It can be cultivated readily.

WHAT IS HARVESTED AND WHEN: Entire plant, when in flower.

USES: A few summers ago, pet shops in California were suddenly sold out of catnip, usually used in toys for cats. Apparently some young people suspected that if it made cats "high," it might do something for them. The fad died a natural death. In Appalachia, a tea made from the plant is used for treating colds, nervous conditions, stomach ailments, and hives; and dried leaves and stalks are smoked to relieve respiratory ailments. The plant has been used to bring on delayed menstruation. A poultice made of it has been applied to reduce swellings.

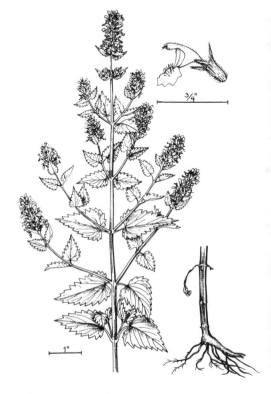

Opuntia spp. Mill.

OTHER COMMON NAME: Indian fig.

PLANT DESCRIPTION: A large cactus growing to 6 feet or more in height, with cylindrical branches and trunk. The spines are ½ to 1½ inches long. The flowers are purple or rose, 2½ inches long. The fruits are green, purple, or brown, finely sticky, and very edible.

WHERE IT GROWS: Dry sunny areas in most of the southern states.

WHAT IS HARVESTED AND WHEN: Roots and stems, as needed; flowers, in early spring.

USES: The stems, which look like flat, spiny green leaves, are roasted and used as a poultice on swellings of all sorts and on the breasts of nursing mothers whose milk supply has dwindled. The roots have been used in an effort to increase hair growth. A tea made of flowers has been drunk to increase urine flow. Indians made tea of the stems and used this as a wash to ease headaches, eye troubles, and insomnia. The early settlers of the West boiled the root in milk and drank the liquid to treat dysentery.

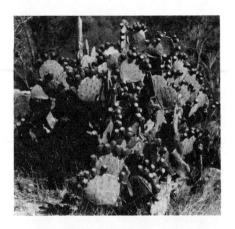

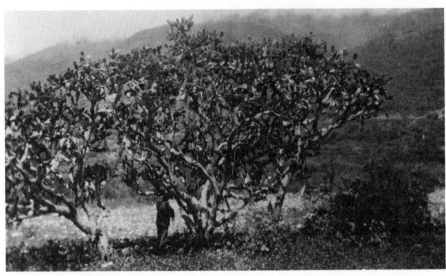

Opuntia tuna Mill.

OTHER COMMON NAME: slipper thorn.

PLANT DESCRIPTION: This succulent plant has no main stem; its flat, leaf-like parts usually have spines. The fruit is pear-shaped and purple and has small spines.

WHERE IT GROWS: Along or near sandy coastal areas and in the deserts of the Southwest. New Mexico, Texas, California, Florida, and elsewhere as a garden escape.

WHAT IS HARVESTED AND WHEN: Fruit, at the end of summer; flat succulent branches, as needed.

USES: In Mexico, the flat branches are scraped clear of spines, cut into small pieces, and used in salads as a vitamin C

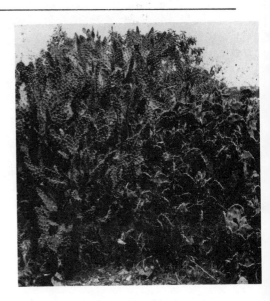

source. The young stems have been boiled in water and applied as a poultice to cure rheumatism. The fruit has been used to treat diarrhea, asthma, and gonorrhea.

Ostrya virginiana (Mill.) K. Koch.

OTHER COMMON NAMES: American hobhorn-beam, deerwood, hardhack, hophornbeam, hornbeam, ironwood, leverwood.

PLANT DESCRIPTION: A tree growing to 60 feet in height. The bark is brown; the leaves are 2 to 5 inches long, slightly fuzzy on both sides, their edges toothed. The fruit clusters are bladder-like, 2 inches long.

WHERE IT GROWS: Lake shores and wooded areas. Eastern United States, from New England south to Florida; west to Texas, Oklahoma, Arkansas, Kansas, Nebraska, the Dakotas, and Minnesota.

WHAT IS HARVESTED AND WHEN: Bark and inner bark, as needed.

USES: The bark has been used both as a laxative and as a tonic. In colonial times,

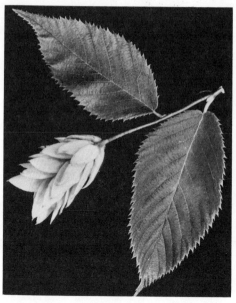 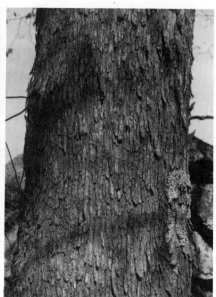

a fluid extract was used to treat malaria. Both bark and inner bark have been used to treat indigestion and fever. A poultice of the bark was once used to reduce swellings of the neck.

VIOLET WOODSORREL   181

Oxalis violacea L.

OTHER COMMON NAMES: jocoyol, shamrock, socoyol, trefoil, woodsorrel.

PLANT DESCRIPTION: A perennial arising from a bulblike base, with flowering stems growing to about 1 foot in height. The leaves consist of three rounded leaflets arising from the basal bulb. The flowers are light purple.

WHERE IT GROWS: Woods, gravelly banks, prairies, and dry upland areas. Eastern United States to Florida; north to Minnesota, Wisconsin, and the Dakotas; west to the Rocky Mountains.

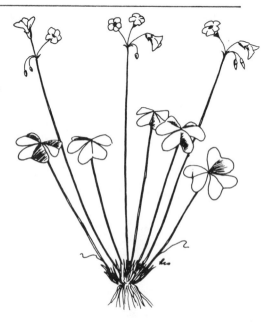

WHAT IS HARVESTED AND WHEN:
Above-ground parts, when plant is in full bloom or later.

USES: In New Mexico, a teaspoonful of fresh or dried powdered leaves is boiled in a cup of water and taken in the morning to help expel intestinal worms. The raw greens have been eaten in the early spring as a blood tonic, after a winter without greens. The plant has been used to create a feeling of coolness in a person with fever, and to increase urine flow.

SOURWOOD   182

Oxydendrum arboreum (L.) DC.

OTHER COMMON NAMES: arrowwood, elk tree, lily of the valley tree, sorrell-tree, sourgum, sourgum bush, titi.

PLANT DESCRIPTION: A tree growing to 50 or 60 feet in height, with deeply fissured bark. The leaves are lance-shaped, 4 to 8 inches long, turning red in the fall. The flowers are white, 1/3 inch long, in drooping clusters 7 to 10 inches long. The fruit is 1/3 inch long, grayish fuzzy, and of varying shapes.

WHERE IT GROWS: Moist or dry woods, well-drained, gravelly soils, and stream banks. Pennsylvania to Indiana, south to Florida and Louisiana, and on the western slopes of the Great Smoky Mountains.

WHAT IS HARVESTED AND WHEN:
Leaves and bark, during growing season.

USES: Indians boiled the leaves and gave feverish patients the liquid to drink; they also used this tea to treat the urinary ailments of older men. A poultice of leaves mixed with bark was used to reduce swellings. The leaves have also been considered a tonic.

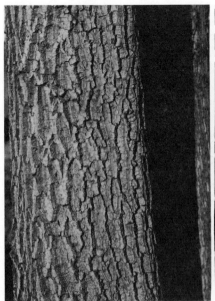
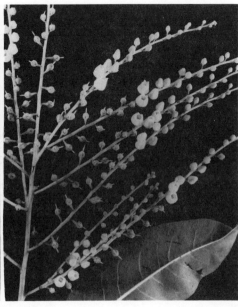

Panax quinquefolius L.

OTHER COMMON NAMES: dwarf groundnut, five fingers, garantogen, garantogere, gensang, ginseng, grantogen, jinshard, manroot, man's health, ninsin, redberry, sang, tartar root.

PLANT DESCRIPTION: A rare perennial with two to four leaves divided into five leaflets at the end of a leafstalk, growing 8 to 10 inches in height. The flowers are small and inconspicuous, the berries vivid, shiny scarlet. The roots are large and aromatic.

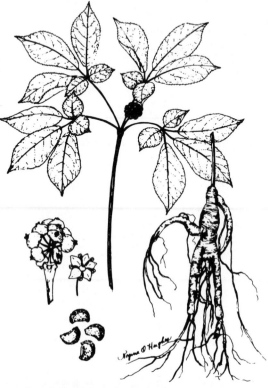

WHERE IT GROWS: Rich, cool woods; in cultivation in shade-houses. New England south to the Appalachian Mountain area to Georgia, west to Oklahoma, Michigan, and Wisconsin.

WHAT IS HARVESTED AND WHEN: Roots from three- to five-year-old plants, in the fall.

USES: This plant has been used by the Chinese for thousands of years, and recent research in Bulgaria, South Korea, and the U.S.S.R. has demonstrated that it is definitely a tonic and stimulant. The Chinese have used the root as an aphrodisiac, and large amounts of the plant are shipped from Appalachia to wherever there are Chinese populations. (At the same time, Korean ginseng is found in American health stores.) In Appalachia, a tea made of the roots is used as a tonic and aphrodisiac. The Indians believed it prevented female conception, and used a root tea to treat rheumatism and vomiting. The root has been used to treat convulsions, dizziness, nervous disorders, colds, fevers, headaches, and shortness of breath, as well as to stop the flow of blood from wounds.

Passiflora incarnata L.

OTHER COMMON NAMES: apricot vine, may pop, maypop herb, passion-flower, passion vine.

PLANT DESCRIPTION: A vine that grows to 30 feet in length. The leaves are alternate, composed of three to five finely toothed lobes. The flowers are showy, 2 inches across, with vivid purple and flesh coloring. The fruit, 2 to 3 inches long, is smooth, yellow, and ovate.

WHERE IT GROWS: Partially shaded dry areas, thickets, fence lines, and edges of wooded areas. Florida west to Texas, north to West Virginia, Maryland, Pennsylvania, Ohio, Indiana, Illinois, and Missouri, and west to Oklahoma.

WHAT IS HARVESTED AND WHEN: Leaves, flowering tops, fruit, and entire plant, during the growing season.

USES: The Indians used the crushed leaves as a poultice to treat bruises and injuries. The fruit juice has been used for sore eyes. The crushed plant tops were used to treat hemorrhoids, burns, and skin eruptions. The plant is reputed to be an aphrodisiac. In Bermuda, the vine is used as a perfume base.

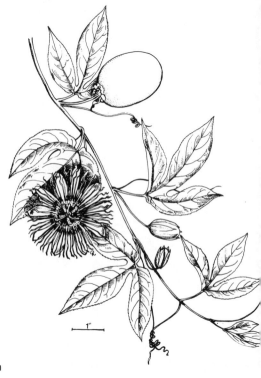

Penstemon pallidus Small

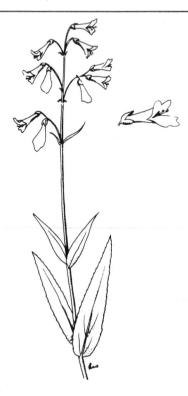

OTHER COMMON NAMES: beard tongue, pentstemon.

PLANT DESCRIPTION: A perennial growing to 3 feet in height, with white flowers. The leaves may have barely visible teeth.

WHERE IT GROWS: Sandy or loamy woods, roadsides, and old fields. New England, west to Michigan, south to Tennessee, Georgia, and Arkansas.

WHAT IS HARVESTED AND WHEN: Roots, as needed.

USES: Indians chewed the root and put the pulp into painful tooth cavities. The root has been used to treat rattlesnake bites and to hasten the movement of the afterbirth from a woman who has delivered a child.

POKEWEED   186

Phytolacca americana L.

OTHER COMMON NAMES: American nightshade, cancer jalap, cancerroot, chongras, coakum, cocum, cokan, common pokeberry, crowberry, garget, inkberry, jalap, pigeonberry, pocan, pocan bush, poke, pokeberry, pokeroot, red-ink plant, red wood, scoke, skoke, Virginia poke.

PLANT DESCRIPTION: A perennial that grows to 9 feet in height and has an extensive system of gnarled roots. The most notable parts of the plant are clusters of dark purple berries that remain well into the winter. The flowers are white to pinkish, borne in terminal clusters.

WHERE IT GROWS: Rich, low ground, field borders, recently cleared areas, roadsides, and abandoned strip-mine areas.

New England, New York, south to Florida and Texas.

WHAT IS HARVESTED AND WHEN:
Very young green leaves, in early spring; roots and berries, in the fall.

USES: Indians used the powdered roots in a poultice to treat cancer. They also applied the roots to the palms and soles of a person with fever. Early settlers used the juice of the berries to treat skin eruptions and cancerous skin ulcers. Dried leaves have been used in poultices on wounds, swellings, and ulcers, and fresh leaves in poultices on old scabs. People in Appalachia not only eat the fresh young green leaves but can them for future use. The plant can be poisonous when mature.

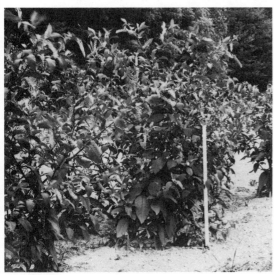

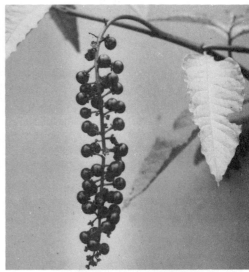

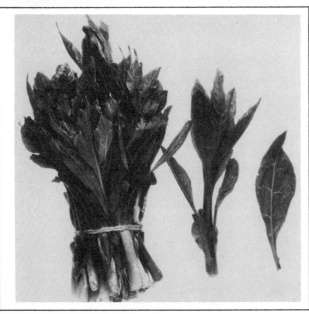

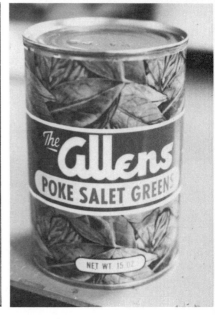

BLACK SPRUCE   187

Picea mariana (Mill.) BSP. *(P. brevifolia, P. nigra, P. abies).*

OTHER COMMON NAMES: bay spruce, blue spruce, double spruce, eastern spruce, he balsam, juniper, shortleaf black spruce, shortleaf spruce, spruce, spruce pine, swamp spruce, water spruce, white spruce, yew pine.

PLANT DESCRIPTION: This abundant evergreen grows to a height of 90 feet on good sites, but in its northern range may reach only 10 to 20 feet, even when 100 to 200 years old. The bark is grayish brown. The cones are short, rounded, ½ to 1½ inches long, purple turning to dull grayish brown. The branches are drooping, brown, and fuzzy. The needles are stiff, crowded, four-sided, somewhat curved, pale blue-green, ¼ to ½ inch long.

WHERE IT GROWS: Well-drained bottomlands and slopes of barren, rocky hills, bogs, and swamps and their borders. New England and the Northeast, west and north to Alaska; around the Great Lakes, including Minnesota, Wisconsin, and Michigan; south from Pennsylvania to Virginia.

WHAT IS HARVESTED AND WHEN: Resin, as needed and available; twigs and cones, at any time; inner bark, most useful in early spring, but can be harvested at any time during the growing season.

USES: A tea made of the inner bark has been used for stomach distress, kidney stones, and rheumatism. The powdered resin has been used on wounds to hasten healing. Indians boiled the twigs and cones in maple syrup to make a beer rich in vitamin C.

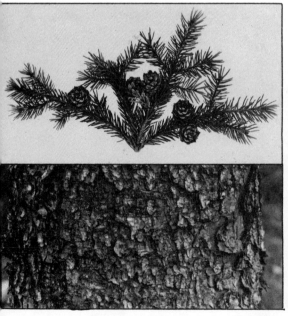

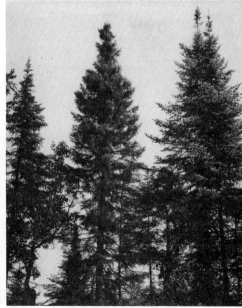

RED SPRUCE   188

Picea rubens Sarg.

OTHER COMMON NAME: he balsam.

PLANT DESCRIPTION: An evergreen
that grows to 100 feet in height. The
bark is reddish, the needles quadrangu-
lar, ½ inch long. The cones are reddish
brown, shiny, oblong, 1½ inches long.

WHERE IT GROWS: Rocky woods and
hillsides, especially in the mountains.
New England south to the western highlands of North Carolina.

WHAT IS HARVESTED AND WHEN:
The pitch, as available.

USES: The pitch was applied to rheumatic joints and to the chest or stomach to
allay pains and discomfort.

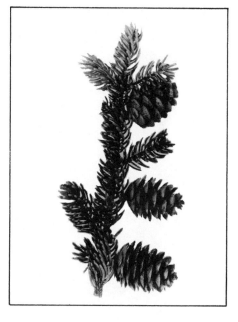

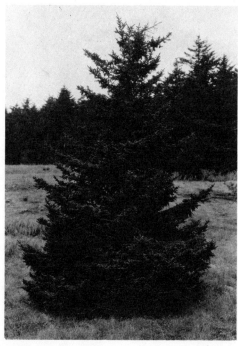

Pinus edulis Engelm. *(P. cembroides* Zucc.)

OTHER COMMON NAMES: Colorado pinyon pine, nut pine, piñon.

PLANT DESCRIPTION: An evergreen tree growing to 40 or 50 feet in height, with short, erect branches forming a narrow head. The branchlets are orange-colored during the first and second year of growth, then become light gray, brown, or reddish tinged. The rigid, triangular, stout needles grow in clusters of two or rarely three.

WHERE IT GROWS: Semiarid and semidesert areas and in alkaline soils. New

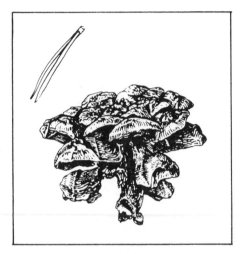

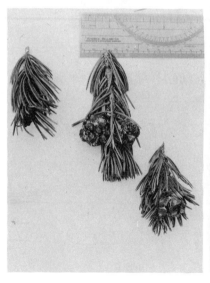

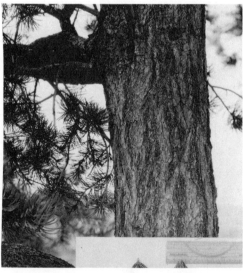

Mexico, Arizona, Colorado, Utah, Oklahoma, Texas, Wyoming, and California.

WHAT IS HARVESTED AND WHEN:
Nuts, in the fall when ripe; needles, as needed; wood, as needed for charcoal, in the fall; resin, as available.

USES: Indians used the charcoal, wrapped in a wet cloth, as a throat compress for laryngitis. California Indians chewed the gum, or resin, for sore throat. They used heated resin to bring boils to a head and to treat sores, insect bites, swellings, and cuts. Hot resin smeared on a warmed cloth was used as a poultice to treat muscular pains, soreness, and pneumonia. Spanish-speaking New Mexicans boil the needles in water, mix the liquid with brown sugar, and drink it as

a remedy for syphilis. The nuts have become popular in recent years as a health food and are sold under the name "pignolia nuts."

LONGLEAF PINE   190

Pinus palustris Mill.

OTHER COMMON NAMES: balsam pine, brown pine, fat pine, Georgia pine, hard pine, heart pine, longleaf yellow pine, longleaved pine, long-leaved pitch pine, longstraw pine, pitch pine, rosemary pine, southern hard pine, southern heart pine, southern pitch pine, southern yellow pine, turpentine pine, yellow pine.

PLANT DESCRIPTION: A majestic evergreen that grows to over 100 feet in height, with coarse, scaly bark. The needles are 8 to 18 inches long, in clusters of three. The cones are 6 to 10 inches long

and cylindrical. Needles are extremely thick on the branches of young trees.

WHERE IT GROWS: This pine prefers sandy soils, and is found from Virginia south to Florida, along the Gulf Coast to the area east of the Mississippi River, northward in Alabama to the foothills of the Appalachian Mountains, Mississippi, Louisiana, and Texas.

WHAT IS HARVESTED AND WHEN: Sap, turpentine, and gum, in early spring.

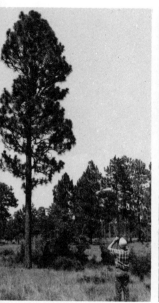 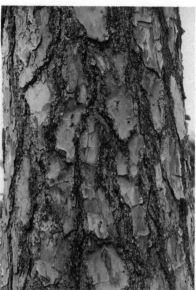 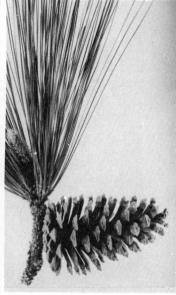

USES: Turpentine, harvested from this tree, is a liquid that solidifies upon exposure. Turpentine oil has been used to treat colic, chronic diarrhea, and tapeworm; applied to a tooth socket, it has been reported to stop bleeding. As an enema, the oil has been used in treating obstinate constipation. The gum has been used to treat kidney ailments and tuberculosis, and to increase or hasten menstrual flow. An application of the solid gum has been applied to surface tumors.

EASTERN WHITE PINE 191

Pinus strobus L.

OTHER COMMON NAMES: American deal pine, American white pine, New England pine, northern pine, northern white pine, soft deal-pine, soft pine, spruce pine, Weymouth pine, white pine.

PLANT DESCRIPTION: These long-lived pines can grow to great heights, and trees 150 feet tall were not uncommon in the virgin forests of Michigan, Pennsylvania, and New England. The branches are dense and horizontal. The needles are soft and bluish green, 3 to 5 inches long, occurring in groups of five. The cones are 4 to 8 inches long, thin, cigar-shaped, yellow-brown, with rounded scales. The bark is thin, smooth, and dark green on young trees and stems, thick and deeply ridged on old trunks.

WHERE IT GROWS: A wide range of habitats from woods and old fields to the banks of streams, on sandy soils as

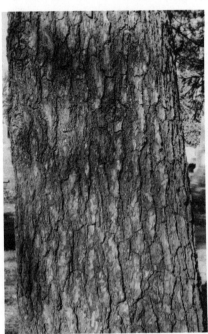
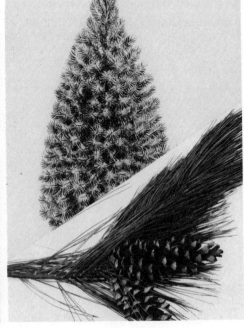

well as fertile, well-drained soils. Eastern North America from Newfoundland to Manitoba; south to Pennsylvania, Ohio, Indiana, Illinois, and Iowa; and southward along the Appalachian Mountains to northern Georgia.

WHAT IS HARVESTED AND WHEN:
Inner bark, during growing season; buds, in early spring; gum and tar, as available.

USES: The bark is used in cough reme-

dies, and has been considered effective both as an expectorant and for reducing swollen tissues. Indians soaked the bark in water until it became soft and then applied it to wounds of all sorts. They also boiled the inner bark of saplings and drank the liquid for dysentery. The gum was applied externally to treat rheumatism and muscular pains. A decoction of the buds is laxative. The tar was used to treat burns and itching, and as a syrup for coughs.

LOBLOLLY PINE 192

Pinus taeda L.

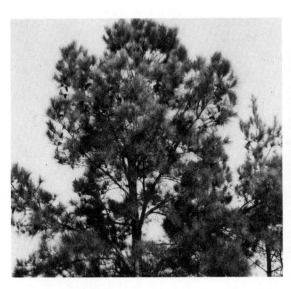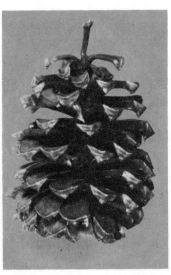

OTHER COMMON NAMES: bastard pine, black pine, bog pine, buckskin pine, bullpine, cornstalk pine, foxtail pine, heart pine, Indian pine, lobby pine, longleaf pine, longschat pine, longschucks, longstraw pine, maiden pine, meadow pine, North Carolina pine, prop pine,

rosemary pine, sap pine, shortleaf pine, slash pine, spruce pine, yellow pine.

PLANT DESCRIPTION: An evergreen tree growing to 100 feet in height. The bright red-brown bark is divided into broad, flat plates covered with large, thin scales. The needles, which occur in bundles of three, are slightly twisted, 6 to 9 inches long. The cones are 2 to 6 inches long, stemless, with short, fat prickles on the scales.

WHERE IT GROWS: Wet clay soils and sandy soils. New Jersey south through Maryland, North and South Carolina, Georgia, Mississippi, the Gulf states, Arkansas, Texas, and Oklahoma.

WHAT IS COLLECTED AND WHEN:
In the winter, people bored holes in the trunks of the trees, and in the spring the borings slowly filled with crude turpentine. The crude material has been separated by distillation into rosin and turpentine oil.

USES: Tar from this tree has been used in a vapor inhaled by persons with pulmonary diseases, and also applied as a salve for skin diseases and blemishes. Oil of turpentine has been used to control intestinal worms, increase urine flow, as a stimulant, and as a laxative.

PLANTAIN   193

Plantago L. spp.

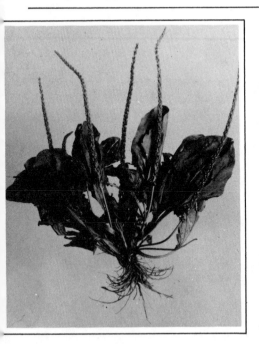

OTHER COMMON NAMES: black psyllium, blond psyllium, fleasweed, French psyllium, Indian plantago, plantago, psyllium, psyllium seed, ribgrass, ribwort, Spanish psyllium.

PLANT DESCRIPTION: A low perennial with broad leaves. The flowers grow at the apex of erect spikes.

WHERE IT GROWS: In poor soils along roadsides and in fields, lawns, and the edges of woods. Throughout the United States.

WHAT IS HARVESTED AND WHEN:
Seeds, in late summer; leaves, as they mature; roots, as needed.

USES: In Appalachia, the leaves are used to make a tea considered a fine tonic. The seeds are a bulk laxative. Soaking the seeds in water causes them to exude a clear, sticky gum which has been used in lotions and wave-set solutions. The leaves have been crushed and bound to bruised parts of the body to reduce swelling. Fresh plantain roots or fresh leaves boiled in water were applied to sore nipples. The plant parts have been used to treat dysentery, extreme constipation, and blood disorders.

Podophyllum peltatum L.

OTHER COMMON NAMES: devil's apple, duck's foot, ground lemon, hog apple, Indian apple, mandrake, mayapple, podophyllum, raccoonberry, umbrella plant, vegetable calomel, vegetable mercury, wild jalap, wild lemon, wild mandrake, yellowberry.

PLANT DESCRIPTION: An erect perennial that grows to 1½ feet in height. It has a single stalk, often forked, with two umbrella-like leaves at the top of the plant. A white flower, 1½ inches across, appears in the fork of the stem, followed by a plumlike yellow fruit.

WHERE IT GROWS: It prefers shady, moist, forested areas but will grow in open glades. New England to Minnesota, and south to Florida and Texas.

WHAT IS HARVESTED AND WHEN: Rootstocks, in the fall or spring.

USES: A resin from the plant has been used to treat warts, and exhibits antitumor properties. In Appalachia, a tea made from the roots is used to treat constipation. The roots have been used to treat jaundice, fever, cancer, liver ailments, and syphilis.

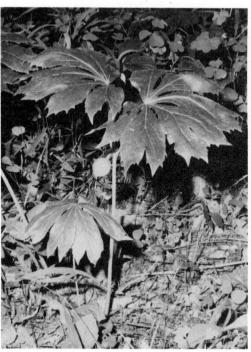
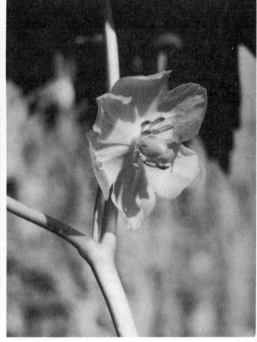

Polygala senega L.

OTHER COMMON NAMES: milkwort, mountain flax, rattlesnake root, seneca-root, seneca snakeroot polygala, senega root, senega snakeroot, seneka snake-root.

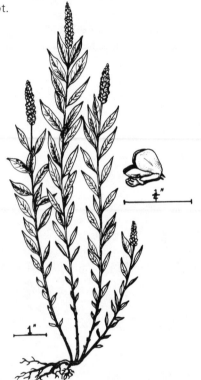

PLANT DESCRIPTION: A perennial that grows to 2½ feet in height, with several stems and narrow, alternate leaves. The crowded spikes of flowers, pink to white with tinges of green, arise at the top of the stem.

WHERE IT GROWS: Dry rocky and gravelly areas and dry woods on rocky soils at higher altitudes. New England to Tennessee, Georgia, and Arkansas, and west to the Dakotas.

WHAT IS HARVESTED AND WHEN: Roots, in the fall; knotty crown, removed when needed.

USES: Indians believed the root was a cure for poisonous snakebites. It was reputed to cure gout, pleurisy, rheumatism, hives, and croup and was also used to treat heart disease. In the 1800's, it received great acclaim as a treatment for pneumonia and other pulmonary infections. In addition, it was believed to be useful as a laxative, to increase urine flow, to produce vomiting, and to treat uterine disorders.

SMALL SOLOMONSEAL   196

Polygonatum biflorum (Walt.) Ell.

OTHER COMMON NAMES: conquer-john, dwarf solomon's seal, hairy solomon's seal, sealwort, solomon's seal.

PLANT DESCRIPTION: A perennial that grows to 3 feet in height. It can be distinguished from the False Solomon's Seal by the fact that its flowers hang from the axils of the leaves. The leaves are 4 inches long, 2 inches wide, and hairy below. The dark blue fruits are globular.

WHERE IT GROWS: Moist, shady woods, hillsides, and thickets. Connecticut and New York south throughout Appalachia to Florida and Texas; west to Michigan, Illinois, Iowa, and Nebraska.

WHAT IS HARVESTED AND WHEN: Roots, in the fall.

USES: A decoction of the roots has been used to treat poison ivy rash and other skin irritations. A liquid made from roots boiled in milk has been drunk to treat hemorrhoids, to serve as a mild laxative, and to increase perspiration. The roots have also been used to reduce pain in the joints caused by arthritis and rheumatism.

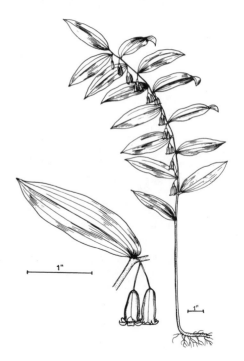

MARSHPEPPER SMARTWEED 197

Polygonum hydropiper L.

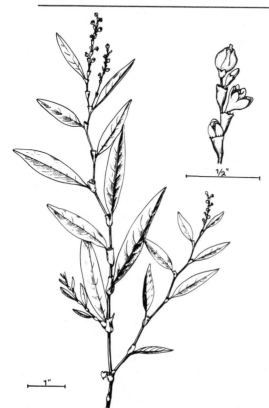

OTHER COMMON NAMES: arsmart, biting knotweed, biting parsicaria, biting tongue, common smartweed, doorweed, lakeweed, pepperplant, red knees, red shanks, red sharks, sickleweed, smartweed, water pepper, water smartweed.

PLANT DESCRIPTION: An erect annual that grows to 2 feet in height. The stems are reddish, and the leaves narrow and alternate, up to 4 inches long, with smooth margins. Small, green flowers are produced close together on the ends of terminal spikes.

WHERE IT GROWS: Damp soils and wet places. Throughout the United States.

WHAT IS HARVESTED AND WHEN: Entire plant, at full bloom.

USES: Dried leaves and tops were boiled in water to make a wash used for sore mouth in nursing mothers. As a medicine, the plant was used for internal bleeding and uterine disorders, and to promote menstrual flow.

NARROWLEAF POPLAR   198

Populus angustifolia James

OTHER COMMON NAMES: alamo sauco, cottonwood, mountain cottonwood.

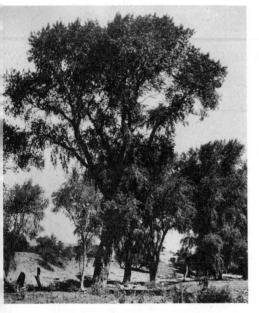

PLANT DESCRIPTION: A tree often growing to 60 feet in height, with a narrow, pyramidal crown. The leaves are narrow, with wavy margins. The bark is greenish.

WHERE IT GROWS: In canyons, along watercourses, on flood plains and stream banks. Dakotas to Nebraska, Wyoming, Montana, Idaho, Nevada, Utah, Arizona, and New Mexico.

WHAT IS HARVESTED AND WHEN: Fruits and flowers, as they ripen.

USES: The cottony flower is dipped in water and placed on an infected gum or tooth. A decoction of the ripe fruit has also been used for toothache. A decoction of the fresh flowers has been used to stop internal hemorrhage. In the spring, a tea of the fresh flowers has been drunk to purify the blood.

BALSAM POPLAR 199

Populus balsamifera L.

OTHER COMMON NAMES: balm buds, balm of Gilead, balsam, black poplar, Carolina poplar, cottonwood, hackmatack poplar, poplar balsam, rough barked poplar, tacamahac, tacamahac poplar, tackamahac.

PLANT DESCRIPTION: A graceful tree that may reach 100 feet in height, with a heavy trunk sometimes 6 feet in diameter. The pointed leaves are 3 to 6 inches long and 2 to 4 inches wide, rounded or heart-shaped at the base, finely toothed, pale green below and shiny dark green above. The large buds are aromatic.

WHERE IT GROWS: Wet woods, swamps, river bottoms, riverbanks, and waste places. All through the Northeast as far south as Maryland and Mississippi; west to Indiana, Iowa, Michigan, Nebraska, Nevada, and Oregon.

WHAT IS HARVESTED AND WHEN: Leaves, as they mature; bark, when needed, winter buds, in February to March, before opening; flowers, in spring.

USES: The fresh flowers and buds are steeped in cold water and strained off; then the liquid is drunk to purify the blood. The leaves and bark have been boiled in water and the vapors inhaled to treat snakebite. Indians boiled the bark and poured the liquid over a broken limb before applying a splint. A bark tincture has been used in treating pulmonary ailments, stomach and kidney disorders, gout, rheumatism, and scurvy.

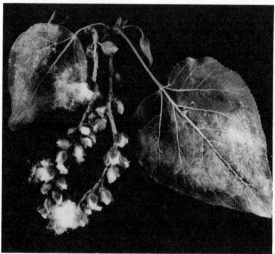
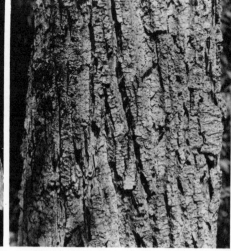

Populus wislizenii (Wats.) Sarg.

OTHER COMMON NAMES: alamo de hoja redonda, cottonwood.

PLANT DESCRIPTION: A tree growing to 45 feet in height, with gray bark and yellowish branches. The leaves are triangular, leathery, toothed, yellow-green, 2½ inches long and 3 inches wide.

WHERE IT GROWS: Along streams and in arroyos, near water holes. Colorado and Texas to Arizona and New Mexico.

WHAT IS HARVESTED AND WHEN: Leaves, when mature; inner bark, in spring or fall.

USES: The inner bark has been used to treat vitamin C deficiency. A decoction of the bark has been used as a wash for bruises and cuts, and a poultice of the boiled bark has been used for treating boils. The boiled leaves were the source of a drink used for curing excess water retention in the body.

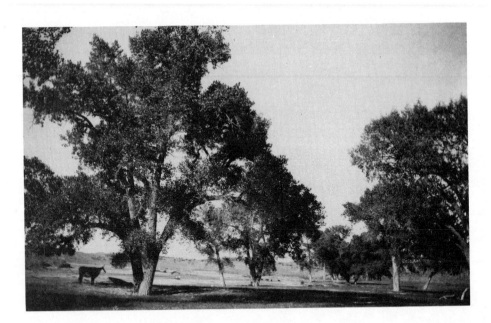

Prosopis glandulosa Torr.

OTHER COMMON NAMES: honey locust, honey mesquite, velvet mesquite.

PLANT DESCRIPTION: A thorny shrub or tree growing to 30 feet in height. The flowers are greenish yellow, occurring in spikes up to 3 inches long. The fruit is a pod, 2 to 7 inches long and about ½ inch broad.

WHERE IT GROWS: Canyons, plains, desert areas, and washes. Southern California, Utah, Colorado, Texas, and Louisiana.

WHAT IS HARVESTED AND WHEN: Leaves, at any time during the growing season; roots, in spring or fall; inner bark in spring and early summer or as needed; gum, when available.

USES: Indians of the Southwest, and the Aztecs, made an eye lotion of the leaves. Other Indians ground the leaves to a powder, wrapped it in a cloth, dampened it, and squeezed the liquid into sore eyes. A root tea was used to treat umbilical hernia in children. Some Indians pounded the white inner bark, boiled it in salt water, and used the drink for indigestion. The boiled sap was used to treat adolescents' skin eruptions. The gummy material was dissolved in water to treat sore throat.

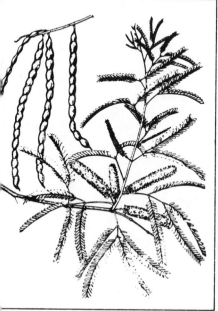

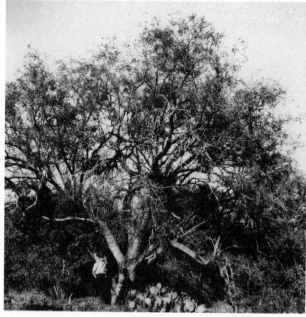

Prunella vulgaris L.

OTHER COMMON NAMES: blue curls, brownwort, carpenter's herb, carpenterweed, common selfheal, dragonhead, hookweed, self-heal, sickleweed, sicklewort.

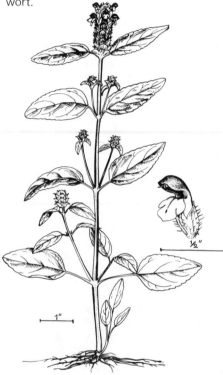

½"

1"

PLANT DESCRIPTION: A perennial that grows to 2 feet in height, though sometimes horizontal. Usually the plant is much tufted, and the leaves are round and bractlike. Violet-purple flowers, about ½ inch long, are found in the axils of the leaves, in a close spike or head.

WHERE IT GROWS: Roadsides, lawns, fields, pastures, wastelands, grasslands, stream banks, and margins of moist woods. Widely distributed in almost all parts of the United States: North Carolina and Kentucky to Florida and Louisiana, Tennessee, Missouri, Kansas, New Mexico, Arizona, and California.

WHAT IS HARVESTED AND WHEN: Flowers and leaves, in summer; entire plant, at full bloom.

USES: This highly aromatic herb has been used to relieve gas and colic. An infusion of the leaves and flowers has been used as a gargle for sore throat and throat irritations, hemorrhages, and diarrhea.

BLACK CHERRY   203

Prunus serotina Ehrh.

OTHER COMMON NAMES: black choke, cabinet cherry, cherry, choke cherry, cokecherry, mountain black cherry, rum cherry, Virginia prune bark, whiskey cherry, wild black cherry, wild cherry.

PLANT DESCRIPTION: A tall tree with a straight trunk, often growing to 100 feet in height. The dark black bark is aromatic. The leaves are shiny, smooth, 2 to 5 inches long, with finely serrated edges. Long, drooping clusters of white flowers are followed by clusters of round, black, bitter-tasting cherries.

WHERE IT GROWS: In a wide range of habitats from streamsides, pastures, and dry woods to wastelands, roadsides, fence rows, and areas near the ocean.

Throughout the eastern states; West Virginia to Georgia, Alabama to Florida; west to Texas, Arizona, and Oklahoma; north to South Dakota and the Lake Superior region.

WHAT IS HARVESTED AND WHEN: Bark, at any time; fruits, in late summer or fall when they have ripened.

USES: In Appalachia, a bark tea is used to treat coughs, colds, and measles. A warm tea was given to women in childbirth and was also used to relieve pains and muscular soreness. An infusion of dried and pulverized berries has been used to treat diarrhea. The pioneers used the bark to treat fever, intestinal worms, indigestion, and tuberculosis. It is considered a useful expectorant.

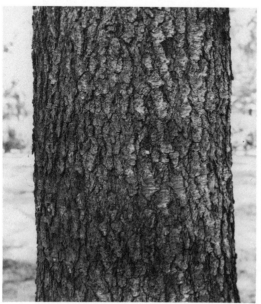
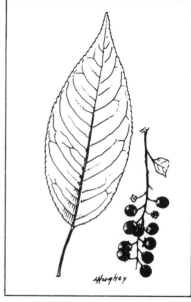

Prunus virginiana L.

OTHER COMMON NAMES: cerisier, chokecherry, western chokecherry, wild cherry.

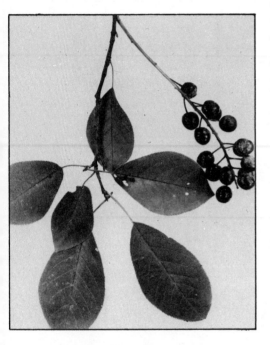

PLANT DESCRIPTION: A tree growing to a height of 20 to 30 feet, with a straight trunk; may be stunted to 3 feet or less in its northern habitat. The bark, which has a disagreeable smell, is fissured to form small scales, often marked by exudations. The leaves at maturity are dark green and shiny above, pale green on the lower surface. The fruit is scarlet or nearly black, round or elongated, and about ¼ inch in diameter.

WHAT IS HARVESTED AND WHEN: Root bark and tree bark, as needed, preferably in the growing season; fruits, in the fall; leaves, as available.

USES: A tea made from the bark, leaves, and dried root has been used for lung ailments and colds. The dried ground bark has been smoked as a treatment for headache and colds, and used as a powder to dry open sores. In Appalachia, a bark tea was used to treat measles and colds. Indians used a warm infusion of the bark to ease the pains of childbirth, and a tea made of the root bark as a sedative and stomach remedy. Early settlers used root bark to treat malaria, worms, tuberculosis, indigestion, and fever. The fruit was sometimes made into a crude wine, which was drunk to relieve dysentery. Hemorrhoids were treated by some Indians with a rectal douche made of boiled bark water.

Pteridium aquilinum (L.) Kuhn

OTHER COMMON NAMES: brake, hog-brake, pasturebrake, western bracken, western brake-fern.

PLANT DESCRIPTION: This fern, with dull green fronds, is 8 to 24 inches in height, stiff, reddish at base, and generally triangular in shape. The brown fruiting bodies are found on the under surface of the fronds.

WHERE IT GROWS: Open woods, thickets, burns, clearings, abandoned fields, and dry woods. Throughout the Northeast; south to North Carolina, Tennessee, Florida, and the coastal plains of the Southeast; north and west to New Mexico, Texas, Colorado, Oklahoma, Wyoming, South Dakota, Minnesota, and Michigan.

WHAT IS HARVESTED AND WHEN: Entire plant, at maturity.

USES: An infusion of the plant has been used to expel intestinal worms and treat diarrhea. Indians used it to increase urine flow and to relieve stomach cramps. A tea was given to women with caked breasts.

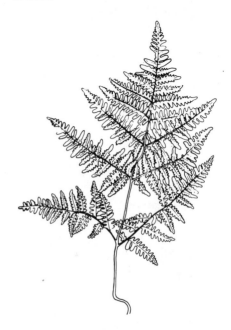

WHITE OAK   206

Quercus alba L.

OTHER COMMON NAMES: common white oak, fork-leaf white oak, ridge white oak, stave oak, stone oak, tanner's oak, West Virginia soft white oak.

PLANT DESCRIPTION: A tree that normally grows from 50 to 75 feet in height, but may reach 150 feet. The bark is light gray, ranging in texture from loosely attached plates or sheets to narrow, rounded ridges with deep fissures on older trees. The leaves are 5 to 9 inches long, smooth, and usually divided into seven to nine smooth, rounded lobes.

WHERE IT GROWS: In hardwood forests, sandy plains, gravelly ridges, well-drained coves, and rich uplands. Throughout the eastern United States, except northern Maine; south to Florida and Mississippi; west to Texas, Oklahoma, Iowa, Kansas, Minnesota; and on the western slopes of the Appalachian Mountains.

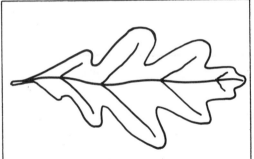

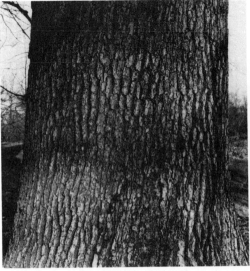

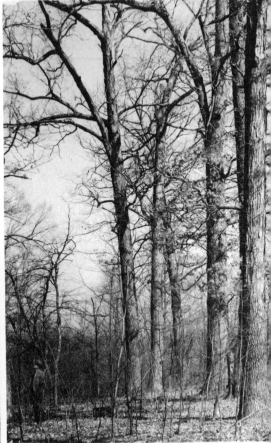

WHAT IS HARVESTED AND WHEN:

Bark, at any time (although bark from older trees is thought to be more useful when harvested in the spring); roots, as needed.

USES: In Appalachia, a tea made from the bark is used to treat burns and sore mouth. The pulverized bark has been used as a substitute for quinine, and a decoction made of boiled bark was used to treat sore eyes. Indians used a tea to treat bleeding hemorrhoids. Roots crushed and mixed with whiskey have been rubbed on rheumatic joints. A root-bark tea has been used to treat gonorrhea and to expel phlegm from the lungs.

GAMBEL OAK   207

Quercus gambelii Nutt.

OTHER COMMON NAMES: encino, encino de la hoja ancha, Gambel's scrub oak, Rocky Mountain white oak, scrub oak.

PLANT DESCRIPTION: A shrub or small tree growing to 45 feet in height. The leaves are 2 to 4 inches long, usually oblong but widest at the tip, with five to nine lobes. The acorns are about ½ inch long, borne in a hemispheric cup.

WHERE IT GROWS: At higher elevations, such as mountains and plateaus. Texas, Arizona, and New Mexico to Colorado, Wyoming, and Utah.

WHAT IS HARVESTED AND WHEN:
Bark and branches, as needed.

USES: Indians used a lotion made from boiled branches, or a powder of the bark, to treat skin sores and skin cancers. A tea made from the bark was drunk to treat diarrhea and malaria.

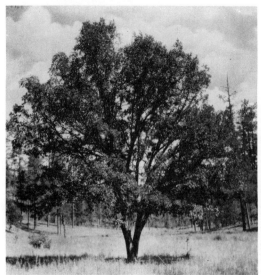
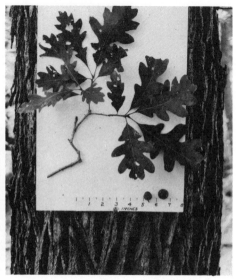

BLACK OAK 208

Quercus velutina Lam.

OTHER COMMON NAMES: black barked oak, dyer's quercus, quercitron, quercitron oak, yellow bark, yellow-barked oak.

PLANT DESCRIPTION: A tree growing to 70 or 80 feet in height, with a trunk up to 4 feet in diameter. The leaves are oblong, usually with seven lobes, dark green above and yellow green below. The inner bark is yellow or orange.

WHERE IT GROWS: Forests and ridges. New England to Florida, west to Texas, north to Nebraska, Minnesota, Michigan, and Illinois.

WHAT IS HARVESTED AND WHEN: Bark, as needed.

USES: Indians crushed the bark and boiled it to make a decoction for treating sore eyes. The bark has been used as a laxative, a tonic, and a treatment for diarrhea, nervous tension, rheumatism, and tuberculosis.

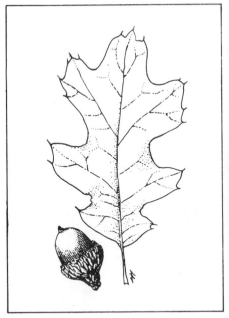

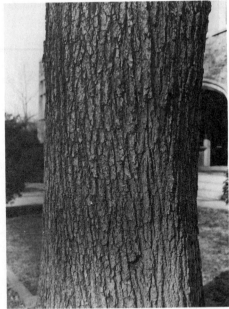

LIVE OAK 209

Quercus virginiana Mill.

OTHER COMMON NAMES: dwarf live oak, green quercus, plateau oak, Rolf's oak, scrub live oak, Virginia live oak.

PLANT DESCRIPTION: An evergreen tree growing to 60 feet in height, with a spreading head and almost horizontal

WHERE IT GROWS: In woods, near the seacoast, on the shores of bays and lakes, near stream banks, on low moist soil, and in wet woods. Virginia, south along the coast of Florida and the Gulf Coast, spreading through Alabama, Louisiana, and Texas.

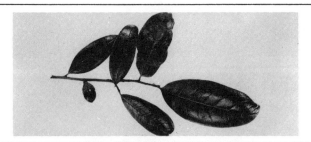

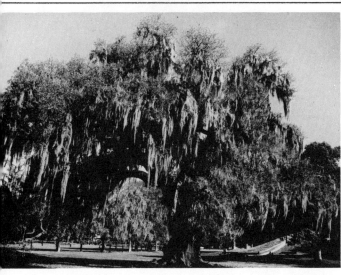

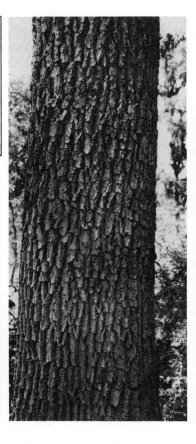

branches. The bark is scaly. The leaves are 1½ to 5 inches long, shiny green above and heavily fuzzy beneath. The acorns are about 1 inch long, the lower fourth enclosed in a woolly cup; one to five in a cluster.

WHAT IS HARVESTED AND WHEN: Bark, as needed.

USES: Indians made a decoction of the crushed bark to treat sore eyes. The bark has also been used to treat dysentery.

Rhamnus purshiana DC.

OTHER COMMON NAMES: bayberry, bearberry, bearwood, bitter bark, buckthorn, California coffee, cascara, cascara sagrada, chittern, chittim, coffee-berry, coffee-tree, Oregon bearwood, shittim, wahoo, western coffee, wild coffee, wild coffee-bush.

PLANT DESCRIPTION: A deciduous tree growing to 25 feet in height. The leaves are 2 to 6 inches long. The flowers are small, greenish yellow, with short stems. The fruit is globular, black, ¼ inch across.

WHERE IT GROWS: Canyon walls, rich bottomlands, along mountain ridges, usually with conifers. Oregon, Washington, California, Idaho, Montana, Colorado, and Arizona.

WHAT IS HARVESTED AND WHEN: Bark, in the fall or spring; fruit, when ripe.

USES: Called the "sacred bark" by early Spanish colonizers, the bark was used by Indians as a laxative and tonic. The berries have been used as a laxative more in Europe than in the United States.

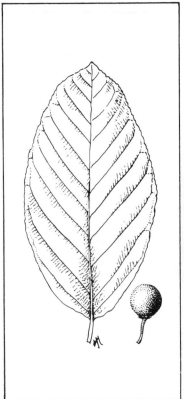
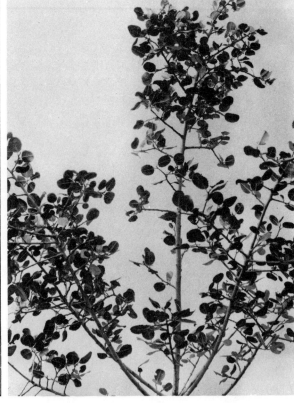

Rhus glabra L.

OTHER COMMON NAMES: common sumac, Pennsylvania sumach, scarlet sumach, shernoke, shoemake, sumac, upland sumach, vinegar tree, white sumach.

PLANT DESCRIPTION: A shrub that grows to 15 feet in height. The leaves are 1 to 3 feet long, composed of up to thirty leaflets; each leaflet is 2 to 4 inches long and about half as wide, pointed and toothed. The greenish yellow flowers are produced in bunches at the ends of branches. The bright red fruits are roundish, flattened, and hairy.

WHERE IT GROWS: Waste areas, margins of woods, old fields, power-line right-of-ways, meadows, and pastures. Arizona and Colorado; eastward to Maine; south to Florida.

WHAT IS HARVESTED AND WHEN: Bark of stem and roots, in spring and fall; ripe fruit, in late summer and early fall; leaves, as needed.

USES: In Appalachia, the leaves are rolled and smoked as a treatment for asthma. The fruits have been used as a refreshing drink and as a gargle for sore throats. The fruits in infusion have been used as a treatment for fever. The bark, boiled in milk, has been used to treat burns. A decoction of bark from stem or roots has been used to treat skin ulcers, gonorrhea, diarrhea, and infections of the lymph glands.

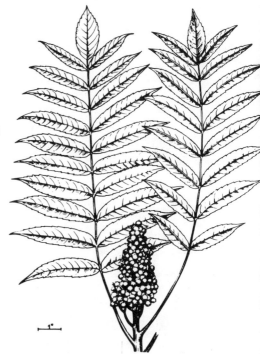

NEW MEXICO LOCUST   212

Robinia neo-mexicana Gray

OTHER COMMON NAME: locust.

PLANT DESCRIPTION: A thorny perennial growing to a height of 25 feet. The leaflets are numerous; the flowers, in dense clusters, fragrant and purple-pink.

WHERE IT GROWS: At elevations of 4,000 to 8,500 feet, in canyons, and in coniferous forests. Southern Colorado to southern Nevada, western Texas, Arizona, and New Mexico.

WHAT IS HARVESTED AND WHEN: Flowers; when mature; foliage, as needed.

USES: Indians used the flowers and the foliage to treat rheumatism and to induce vomiting. Cattle and deer enjoy both foliage and flowers.

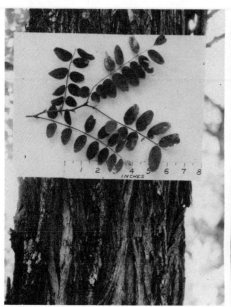
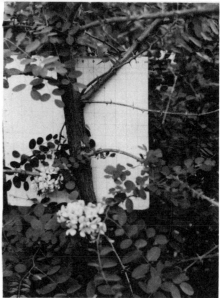

BLACKBERRY   213

Rubus spp. L.

OTHER COMMON NAMES: brambleberry, dewberry, raspberry.

PLANT DESCRIPTION: A shrubby or viny perennial, with thorns, that produces large white flowers. The fruit is either red or black.

WHERE IT GROWS: Old fields, waste areas, forest borders, and pastures. Throughout the United States.

WHAT IS HARVESTED AND WHEN: Roots and root bark, in spring and fall; fruits, in summer as they ripen.

USES: In Appalachia, a tea made from the roots is used to dry up runny noses; a tea made from the root bark, to stop dy-

sentery. The juice of the fruit has been used to control dysentery in children.

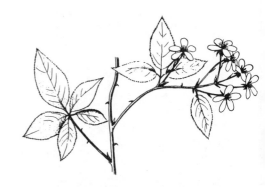

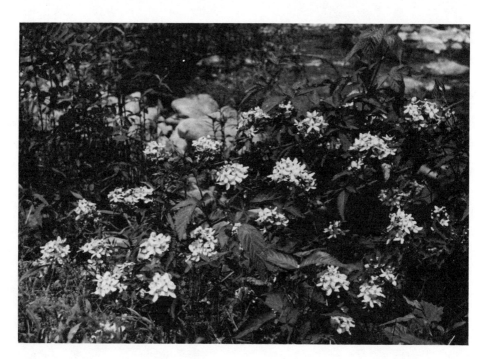

GOLDEN-GLOW   214

Rudbeckia laciniata L.

OTHER COMMON NAMES: cone disk, coneflower, cutleaf coneflower, dormilon, tall coneflower, thimble weed.

PLANT DESCRIPTION: A branching perennial up to 10 feet in height. The stem has short, stiff hairs. The flowers

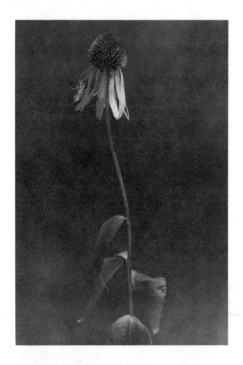

occur in heads, with greenish yellow centers surrounded by yellow rays.

WHERE IT GROWS: Most places, especially stream banks and rich, low fields. New England south to Florida, Louisiana, Texas, Arizona, New Mexico, and Montana.

WHAT IS HARVESTED AND WHEN: Leaves, when mature; entire plant, when in bloom.

USES: New Mexicans make a tea of the green leaves, add pieces of stork's bill (*Erodium cicutarium*) stalk, strain the liquid, and drink it for ten days to cure gonorrhea or induce menstruation. The plant has been used to increase urine flow and to treat kidney trouble and Bright's disease.

CURLY DOCK   215

Rumex crispus L:

OTHER COMMON NAMES: bitter dock, curled dock, dock, garden patience, narrow dock, sour dock, yellow dock.

PLANT DESCRIPTION: A perennial that grows to 5 feet in height. The leaves are narrow, 6 to 12 inches long, with curly edges. The flowers are yellow to green, borne in clusters. The seeds are winged and triangular.

WHERE IT GROWS: Pastures, fields and wastelands, yards, and old building sites. Throughout the United States.

WHAT IS HARVESTED AND WHEN: Roots, when the plant is large enough; leaves, in the summer and early fall.

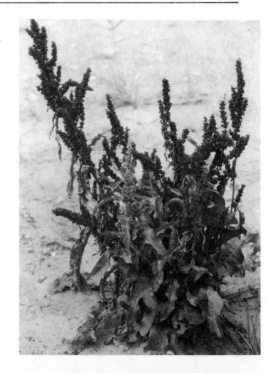

USES: Crushed green leaves were applied to boils to bring them to a head. The juice of the leaves has been used to treat ringworm and other skin parasites. In Appalachia, a wash made of roots soaked in vinegar is still used to treat ringworm, and a poultice made of leaves is used for nervous or allergic hives. Fresh roots boiled in water provide a decoction used internally as a laxative and a treatment for skin ailments.

CANAIGRE 216

Rumex hymenosepalus Torr.

OTHER COMMON NAMES: tanners dock, wild pieplant, wild rhubarb.

PLANT DESCRIPTION: A perennial growing to 3 feet in height. The leaves are sometimes 1 foot long, with sheaths at base of each leaf. The flowers, in clusters, are 6 to 12 inches long and rose-colored. The tubers resemble sweet potatoes.

WHERE IT GROWS: Sandy stream banks, old fields, dry plains, and hillsides. Wyoming to Utah, Texas, Arizona, New Mexico, and California.

WHAT IS HARVESTED AND WHEN: Roots, when one year old or older.

USES: The dried root has been ground into a powder and applied as a poultice for sore joints. A tea made from the roots has been used to treat sore throat and diarrhea.

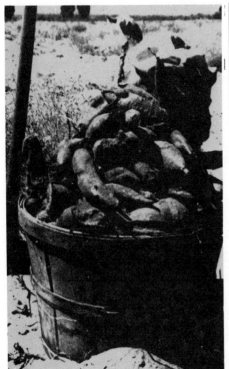

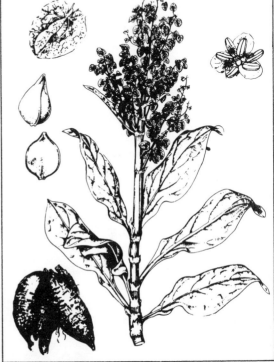

BITTER DOCK   217

Rumex obtusifolius L.

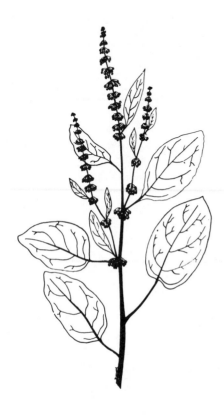

OTHER COMMON NAMES: blunt-leaved dock, broad-leaved dock, common dock, obtuse-leaved rumex, red-veined dock.

PLANT DESCRIPTION: A perennial growing to 4½ feet in height. The lower leaves are 7 to 14 inches long and 3 to 6 inches wide; the upper leaves are narrower. The flowers appear on slender stalks and are greenish or brownish.

WHERE IT GROWS: Fields; waste areas, empty lots, and roadsides. Throughout the United States.

WHAT IS HARVESTED AND WHEN: Roots, as needed.

USES: A decoction of the root has been used externally to treat skin diseases and internally as a laxative. Fresh or dried roots boiled in water have been used as a decoction for treating venereal disease. A poultice of the root has been applied to ulcers, skin itch, and other skin diseases.

COMMON RUE   218

Ruta graveolens L.

OTHER COMMON NAMES: country man's treacle, garden rue, herb-of-grace, ruda.

PLANT DESCRIPTION: A strong-smell-ing annual growing to 3 feet in height, covered with a whitish bloom. The leaves are 2 to 4 inches long. The flowers are ½ inch across, yellowish, with toothed petals.

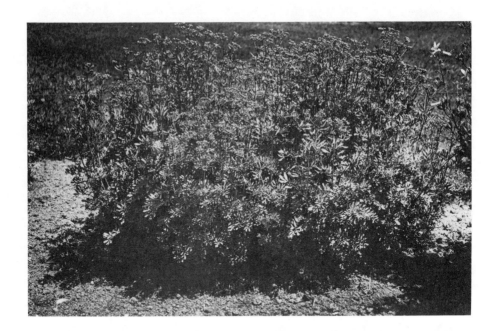

WHERE IT GROWS: Old fields and pastures, roadsides, and waste areas. New England to Florida, west to Texas and Missouri, and in Appalachia.

WHAT IS HARVESTED AND WHEN: Plant, at full bloom; leaves, when mature.

USES: An infusion of the plant has been used to treat stomach gas and colic, epilepsy, and nervous distress; to promote delayed menstruation; and to produce abortions. Indians considered the plant useful for promoting fertility. As a poultice, it has been applied to joints affected by rheumatism. Mixed with tobacco, it has been smoked as a sedative and to treat neuralgia. A leaf tea has been used for indigestion. Leaf juice has been given to children to stop convulsions and fits.

Salix alba L.

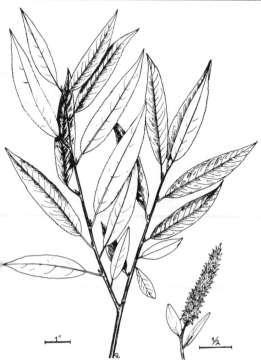

1"   ½

OTHER COMMON NAMES: common willow, European white willow, European willow, Huntington willow.

PLANT DESCRIPTION: An attractive tree that grows to 75 feet in height, with spreading, drooping branches. Young branchlets are silky white, turning dark olive-brown as they mature. The leaves are 1½ to 4 inches long, narrow and pointed, with finely toothed edges, glossy green above and silky white below. The flowers are catkins.

WHERE IT GROWS: Rich, low woods, roadsides, shores, and stream banks. New England, to North Carolina, Virginia, Georgia, Tennessee, Kentucky, and West Virginia.

WHAT IS HARVESTED AND WHEN: Leaves, during the growing season; bark, at any time.

USES: In Appalachia, a tea made of the leaves and bark is used to reduce fever. The bark has been used as a tonic in convalescence, and for treatment of diarrhea and menstrual irregularity.

BLACK WILLOW 220

Salix nigra (Marsh.)

OTHER COMMON NAMES: pussy willow, swamp willow, willow.

PLANT DESCRIPTION: A tree that often grows to 40 feet in height, but may grow much taller. The leaves are narrow, 3 to 6 inches long, ½ to ¾ inch wide, finely toothed, and sharply pointed. The twigs are reddish brown. The flowers are catkins, 1 to 3 inches long.

WHERE IT GROWS: Stream banks, meadows, and rich, low woods. North Dakota and Colorado south to Florida,

Alabama, and Texas and eastward to Tennessee.

WHAT IS HARVESTED AND WHEN:
Bark, with buds, stripped from two- to three-year-old branches in spring, about the time growth begins; catkins, early spring.

USES: Indians used a tea made of bark to treat lumbago, and an infusion of the bark to treat colds and asthma and increase perspiration. They believed the catkins to be aphrodisiac. The bark has been used in a tea to treat indigestion, diarrhea, ulcers, and gangrene.

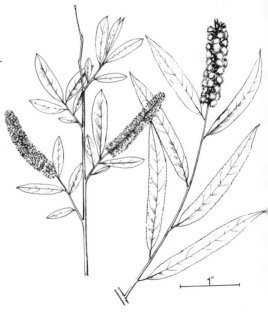

RUSSIAN THISTLE   221

Salsola kali L.

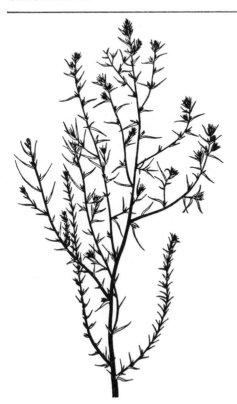

OTHER COMMON NAMES: barilla plant, common saltwort, Russian tumbleweed, saltwort, tumbling thistle.

PLANT DESCRIPTION: An annual, round and bushy, growing to 3 feet in height. The leaves are prickly, pointed, and fuzzy. The flowers are greenish white to pink, small, and solitary, appearing at the apex of branches.

WHERE IT GROWS: Grain regions of the western and plains states, old fields, and seashores. New England to Florida; Midwest, including Ohio, Indiana, Illinois; and to Missouri.

WHAT IS HARVESTED AND WHEN:
Plant, when blooming.

USES: The plant has been used to promote menstrual flow, increase urine flow, and decrease water retention in the body.

Salvia officinalis L.

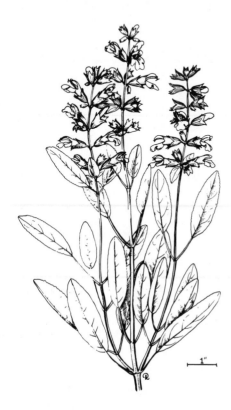

PLANT DESCRIPTION: A fuzzy peren- nial that grows to 3 feet in height. The leaves have toothed edges. The flowers, which grow on terminal spikes in whorls of four to eight, are blue or white.

WHERE IT GROWS: Dumps, waste- lands, old fields, roadsides, and gardens. Throughout the United States.

WHAT IS HARVESTED AND WHEN: Leaves, during flowering.

USES: In the early 1800's, the crushed fresh leaves were thought to have the power to destroy warts. They have been used as an antiseptic, a tonic, and to re- lieve skin wounds and cuts. Indians used a salve of the leaves mixed with grease to treat skin sores. The plant has also been used to treat coughs, colds, night sweats, worms, and (as a gargle) ulcer- ous sore throat. In Appalachia, a tea made from the leaves has been used as a mild laxative and a treatment for stomach gas. In Europe, extracts have been used to reduce the milk flow of mothers at weaning time.

OTHER COMMON NAMES: meadow sage, sage, scarlet sage, true sage.

Sambucus canadensis L.

OTHER COMMON NAMES: common elder, elder, elderberry, sweet elder.

PLANT DESCRIPTION: A shrub grow- ing to 12 feet in height. The branches are yellowish gray; the pith is white. The leaves are made up of leaflets, usu- ally toothed. The flowers are white; the fruit purplish black, ¼ inch in diameter.

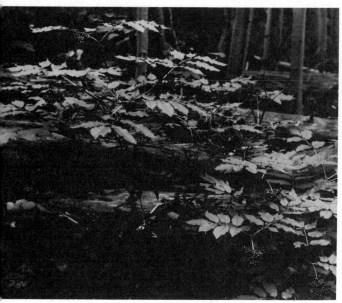 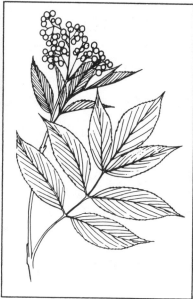

WHERE IT GROWS: Moist soils and woods, roadsides, and fields. New England south to Georgia, Louisiana, and Oklahoma.

WHAT IS HARVESTED AND WHEN: Bark and roots, as needed; fruit and flowers, when available.

USES: The bark was simmered in lard in pioneer times to make a soothing ointment for chafed skin, abrasions, ulcers, and burns. The juice of the root and the boiled bark were used in cases of water retention. The flowers and fruits were made into poultices for treating rheumatism, sores, and burns. The beaten and mashed leaves were used as a poultice for headaches. Indians pounded the smaller roots, stirred them in hot water, and tied them to the swollen breasts of women. The berries were fermented by early settlers to make a tonic wine and a cooling lotion for feverish patients.

BLOODROOT   224

Sanguinaria canadensis L.

OTHER COMMON NAMES: coomroot, pauson, puccoon, puccoon root, red Indian paint, red puccoon, redroot, snakebite, sweet slumber, tetterwort, turmeric, white puccoon.

PLANT DESCRIPTION: A perennial that grows to 6 to 14 inches in height, with a solitary leaf stem. The leaves are palmately lobed around the outer edge. In early spring, conspicuous white flowers are produced, 1 to 2 inches in width. The roots are vivid red.

WHERE IT GROWS: Deep, cool, moist deciduous woods and woodland slopes; rich soils. New England, Long Island, Pennsylvania, New Jersey, Kentucky, Ohio, Indiana, Wisconsin, Illinois, Kansas, Florida to Texas.

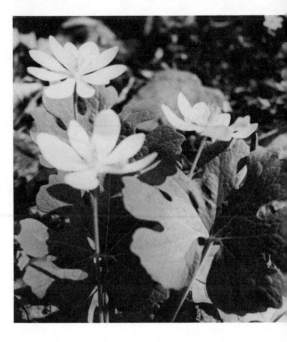

WHAT IS HARVESTED AND WHEN: Roots, during the growing season till late fall.

USES: Captain John Smith reported that the Indian women selected to share his quarters painted themselves red with bloodroot. Indians used the root to induce vomiting, and some used it in religious services to aid in divination. A tea made from the root was used to treat fever and rheumatism; some tribes chewed the root and placed the spittle on skin burns—a dangerous practice because the root is violently toxic. Some New England Indians squeezed juice from the root onto a lump of maple sugar and held it in the mouth to cure sore throat—another risky practice. The root has been used to clear the throat and nasal passages of mucus, as a tonic, and to induce vomiting—also dangerous.

BOUNCINGBET   225

Saponaria officinalis L.

OTHER COMMON NAMES: bruisewort, chimney-pink, common soapwort, crow-soap, Londonpride, sheepweed, wild sweet William, wood-phlox.

PLANT DESCRIPTION: A smooth, erect perennial growing to 2 feet in height. The flowers are in dense clusters, pinkish to white.

WHERE IT GROWS; Along railroad right-of-ways, waste places, and roadsides. New York south to Georgia and as far west as Indiana.

WHAT IS HARVESTED AND WHEN: Roots, in the fall.

USES: Because of its high saponin content (which produces a soapy lather), the plant has been used in washing clothes. The root has been used to treat gout, syphilis, and rheumatism.

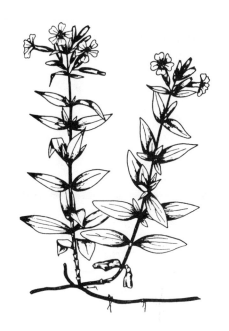

SASSAFRAS   226

Sassafras albidum (Nutt.) Nees.

OTHER COMMON NAMES: ague tree, cinnamon wood, common sassafras, red sassafras, saxifras, smelling stick, white sassafras.

PLANT DESCRIPTION: A tree that grows to 40 feet in height. The leaves are of three different shapes: three-lobed, two-lobed, and mitten-shaped and un-lobed. Fragrant, yellowish green flowers are borne in clusters, male and female flowers usually occurring on different trees. In the fall, the female flowers develop into dark blue, one-seeded berries about pea size, borne on a red stalk.

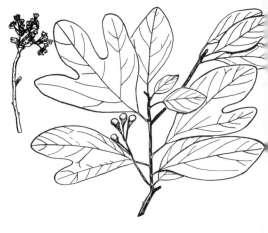

WHERE IT GROWS: Woods, roadsides, thickets, along fence rows, and in aban- doned fields. New England, New York, Ohio, Illinois, and Michigan, south to Florida and Texas.

WHAT IS HARVESTED AND WHEN:
Root bark, in spring and fall.

USES: A tea of the root bark is used in Appalachia to treat bronchitis. It has also been used to increase urine flow, relieve gas and upset stomach, and increase perspiration. In the early 1800's, sassafras tea was used to slow down the milk flow in nursing mothers. The bark has been used as a poultice for sore eyes. The tea has also been used to treat kidney trouble, dysentery, and respiratory ailments.

MARYLAND FIGWORT   227

Scrophularia marilandica L.

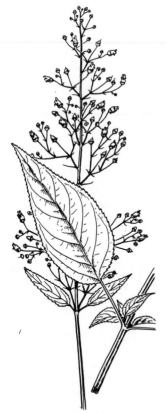

OTHER COMMON NAMES: brownwort, bullwort, carpenter's square, figwort, great pilewort, heal-all, Holme's weed, kernelwort, knotted root, murrian grass, pilewort, scrofula plant, square stalk, stinking Christopher.

PLANT DESCRIPTION: A perennial shrub that grows to 10 feet in height, with four-angled stems. The leaves are 4 to 12 inches long, with toothed margins, thin and tapering to a point. Small, reddish brown flowers are found at the top of the plant.

WHERE IT GROWS: Empty fields, roadsides, forests, and forest openings. Maine to Minnesota; south to South Carolina, Georgia, Alabama, and Louisiana; and west to Oklahoma.

WHAT IS HARVESTED AND WHEN:
Entire plant, at full bloom; roots, in the fall; bark, in the spring and fall.

USES: An infusion of the fresh roots in water was used in the 1800's to treat anxiety, restlessness, and insomnia in pregnant women. A poultice was used to treat skin diseases such as impetigo and cradle cap. The entire plant was used as a tonic, to break a fever by increasing perspiration, to increase urine flow, and to cure intestinal worms. The bark of the plant and the roots were used as treatments for tuberculosis, scabies, and open wounds. The plant was used at various times to increase menstrual flow and treat hemorrhoids.

Scutellaria lateriflora L.

OTHER COMMON NAMES: American skullcap, blue pimpernel, blue skullcap, helmet flower, hooded willow herb, hoodwort, mad-dog, mad-dog skullcap, mad-dog weed, madweed, skullcap.

PLANT DESCRIPTION: An erect perennial that grows to 3 feet in height. The leaves are thin, 1 to 4 inches long, pointed and coarsely toothed. The flowers are blue and arranged along spikes in the upper leaf axils.

WHERE IT GROWS: Moist woods, damp areas, alluvial thickets, meadows, and swampy areas. Throughout the United States.

WHAT IS HARVESTED AND WHEN: Entire plant, in bloom.

USES: At one time, the plant was believed to be a cure for rabies and for

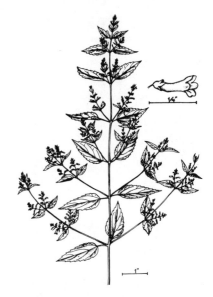

hysteria. Indians used it to help eliminate a mother's afterbirth, to promote menstruation, and to treat diarrhea and heart disease. It has been used as a sedative and to increase perspiration.

Senecio aureus L.

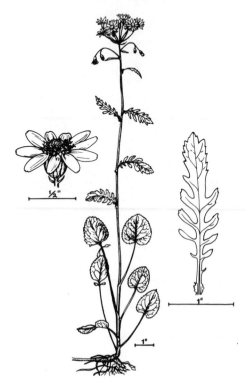

OTHER COMMON NAMES: butterweed, cocashweed, coughweed, false valerian, female regulator, golden groundsel, golden rod, golden senecio, ground-sel, liferoot, life-root plant, ragwort, squawweed, swamp squawweed, uncum, waxweed, wild valerian.

PLANT DESCRIPTION: A perennial that grows to 3 feet in height, with erect flowering stems. The flowers are bright yellow; the roots are mostly horizontal.

WHERE IT GROWS: Moist woods, swampy places, and humid areas. Florida to Texas; north to Maryland, Kentucky, and Missouri; and west to Minnesota and Arkansas.

WHAT IS HARVESTED AND WHEN: Above-ground portions, in full bloom; roots, at the same time or later.

USES: Root and plant have been used interchangeably. Indians made a tea of the flowering plant to relieve the pains of childbirth, to hasten delayed childbirth, and for kidney problems. An infusion of the entire plant in water was used to treat coughs, nervous disorders, weakness due to prolonged fever, and poor circulation.

SAW-PALMETTO 230

Serenoa serrulata (Michx.) Hook

PLANT DESCRIPTION: A low-growing fan palm, sometimes having a trunk, and growing to 20 feet in height. The saw-toothed green leaves are covered with a whitish bloom. The inconspicuous flow-ers appear in branching clusters. The fruit varies in size and shape.

WHERE IT GROWS: Swampy low areas, near coastal regions. South Caro-

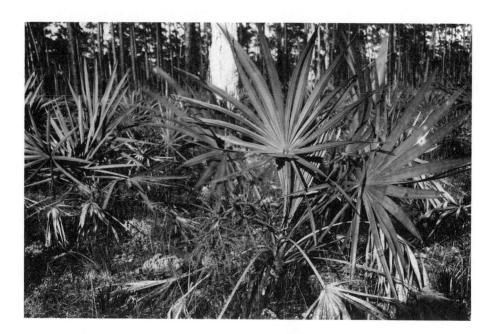

lina to Florida, Mississippi, and coastal Texas.

WHAT IS HARVESTED AND WHEN:
Fruits, when ripe; roots and leaves, as needed; inner bark, spring or summer.

USES: Indians used the seeds for food. They made an infusion of leaves and roots for treating dysentery and relieving stomach pains. They made the inner trunk bark into poultices and applied them to snakebites, insect bites, and skin ulcers. The dried ripe fruits were believed to have sedative properties and to be useful for treating respiratory infections and improving digestion.

FAT SOLOMONPLUME   231

Smilacina amplexicaulis Nutt.

OTHER COMMON NAME: false Solomon's seal.

PLANT DESCRIPTION: A perennial 1 to 3 feet in height. The leaves are 2 to 5 inches long, with a clasping base. The flowers are small, whitish, borne in groups. The fruit is a berry, red with purple dots.

WHERE IT GROWS: In cool, shaded arroyos and ravines, moist and shaded woods, roads, and hillsides. Oregon and Washington to California and New Mexico.

WHAT IS HARVESTED AND WHEN:
Roots, during the growing season; leaves, when large enough.

USES: The smoke of the burning root was used to revive a fainting person. A tea made of the leaves was thought to prevent conception.

231

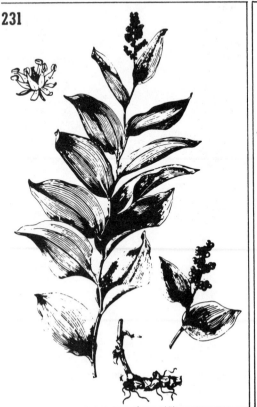

232

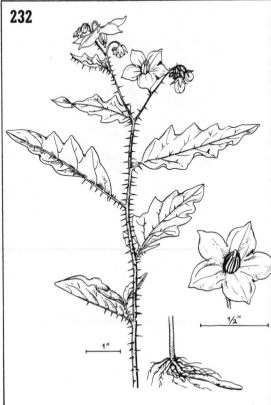

½"

1"

HORSE NETTLE   232

Solanum carolinense L.

OTHER COMMON NAMES: apple of Sodom, ball nettle, bull nettle, Carolina horse nettle, nightshade, sand brier, tread-softly.

PLANT DESCRIPTION: A prickly, straight-growing perennial that grows to 3 feet in height. The leaves have yellow spines on the veins of the lower surface. The flowers are white to light violet.

The fruit is globular, yellow, and ½ inch in diameter.

WHERE IT GROWS: Open fields, roadsides, and waste lands. In most of the United States.

WHAT IS HARVESTED AND WHEN: Berries, leaves, and rootstocks, in the fall.

206

USES: In colonial times, the juice of five or six berries, taken daily in increasing quantities, was used to treat tetanus. The berries have been used to promote urination, relieve pain, and ease nervous tension. The entire plant has been considered useful in treating epilepsy, asthma, bronchitis, and convulsions. The root is believed to be a sedative.

AMERICAN MOUNTAINASH 233

Sorbus americana Marsh.

OTHER COMMON NAMES: American rowan tree, American service tree, dogberry, Indian mozemize, life-of-man, masse-misse, missy-massy, missey-moosey, mountain ash, mountain sumach, quick beam, round tree, roundwood, wild ashe, wine tree, witchwood.

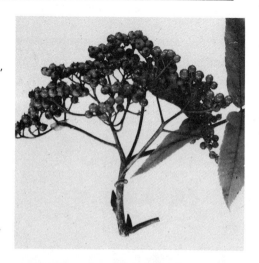

PLANT DESCRIPTION: A small tree that grows to 25 feet in height, with smooth, gray bark. The compound leaves have eleven to seventeen pointed leaflets, with toothed edges. The clusters of white flowers are followed by bright red berries, about ¼ inch in diameter.

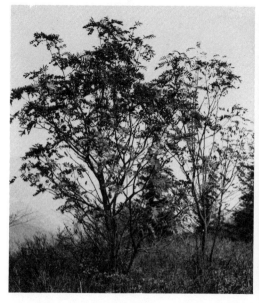

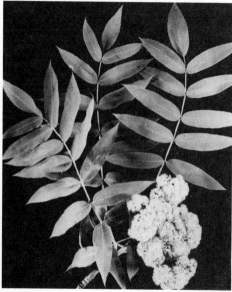

WHERE IT GROWS: Borders of swamps, rocky hillsides, forests, and waste areas. At higher elevations in the northeastern United States, Great Lakes region to Minnesota, from Pennsylvania to West Virginia, North Carolina, and Tennessee, and in the Appalachian Mountains.

WHAT IS HARVESTED AND WHEN:

Bark, as needed; fruits, in the fall.

USES: The berries are rich in vitamin C and have been used, fresh and in tea, to treat scurvy. The bark has been used as a tea for nausea and to cleanse the blood in the spring. The Indians used bark preparations for heart disease.

PINKROOT SPIGELIA   234

Spigelia marilandica L.

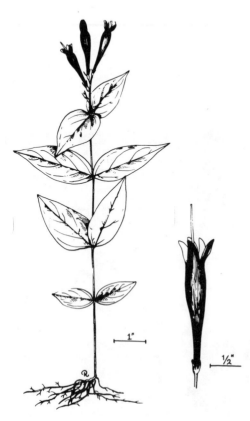

OTHER COMMON NAMES: American wormroot, Carolina pink, Carolina pinkroot, Indian pink, Maryland pinkroot, perennial wormgrass, pinkroot, snakeroot, star bloom, unstilla, wormgrass.

PLANT DESCRIPTION: A perennial that grows to 2 feet in height. The leaves are stemless, lance-shaped. The flowers are red on the outside, yellow on the inside, funnel-shaped, along one side of a flowering spike.

WHERE IT GROWS: Rich woods and thickets. Eastern United States to Florida and Texas.

WHAT IS HARVESTED AND WHEN: Roots, in the fall after flowering; entire plant, at full bloom; leaves, as needed.

USES: In Appalachia, a tea made from the leaves is used to aid digestion. Fresh roots and a tea of the entire plant were used by Indians to treat intestinal worms. A tea made from the root was used to treat malaria.

Spiraea tomentosa L.

OTHER COMMON NAMES: red meadow, silver weed, steeple bush, sweet hardhack, white cap, white leaf.

PLANT DESCRIPTION: A shrub growing to 4 feet in height. The branches are reddish brown and woolly. The leaves, up to 3 inches in length, are woolly beneath, and toothed. The flowers are pinkish, sometimes white.

WHERE IT GROWS: Barren fields, dry meadows, bogs, and old pastures. New England south to South Carolina and Mississippi; Appalachian areas.

WHAT IS HARVESTED AND WHEN: Leaves, as needed; root bark and stems, in spring and fall; flowers, as they appear.

USES: The leaves and bark when boiled in water produce a tea for treating diarrhea. A poultice of the leaves and bark has been applied to tumors and ulcers. Indians made a tea from flowers and leaves, used during pregnancy and to ease childbirth.

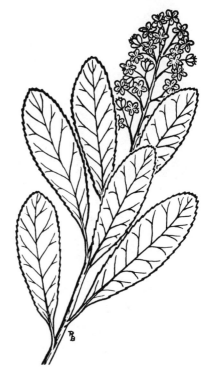

Stellaria media (L.) Cyrillo

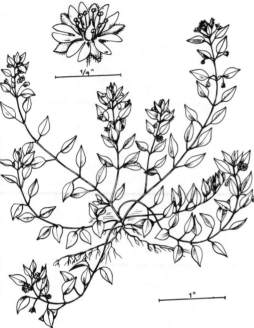

1/4"

1"

OTHER COMMON NAMES: adder's mouth, common chickweed, satin flower, starwort, stitchwort, tongue grass, white bird's eye.

PLANT DESCRIPTION: An annual that grows to 12 to 15 inches in height. The stems are matted to somewhat upright. The upper leaves lack stems and vary in shape; the lower leaves are ovate. The small individual flowers are white.

WHERE IT GROWS: Shaded areas, meadows, dooryards, cultivated ground, waste land, thickets, gardens, and damp woods. Virginia to South Carolina and southeast.

WHAT IS HARVESTED AND WHEN: Entire plant, at full bloom.

USES: A poultice made of the plant has been used to treat skin sores, ulcers, and infections as well as eye infections and hemorrhoids.

Stellaria pubera Michx.

OTHER COMMON NAMES: giant chickweed, great starwort, star chickweed, stitchweed.

PLANT DESCRIPTION: A perennial with a woody base, growing to 18 inches in height. The leaves are ½ to 1½ inches long, with short stalks or none. The flowers are white, about ¼ to ½ inch long.

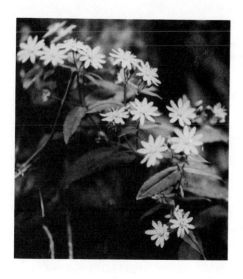

WHERE IT GROWS: Rich, moist woods. New Jersey south to the Appalachian area, Florida, Georgia, Mississippi, and Alabama.

WHAT IS HARVESTED AND WHEN: Juice of the mature plant and the entire plant, when in bloom.

USES: The juice of the plant, high in vitamin C, has been used to treat scurvy. An infusion of the plant has been used for lung congestion and tuberculosis, and as a tonic after illness.

QUEENSDELIGHT   238

Stillingia sylvatica L.

OTHER COMMON NAMES: cock-up-hat, cocyshat, marcony, nettle potato, queen's delight stillingia, queen's root, silver leaf, stillingia, yaw root.

PLANT DESCRIPTION: A milky-juiced perennial that grows to 3 feet in height. The leaves are stemless, leathery, and fleshy. The flowers are yellow.

WHERE IT GROWS: Dry woods, sandy soils, pine barrens, old fields, and forest clearings. Virginia to Florida, Kansas, and Texas; north to Oklahoma.

WHAT IS HARVESTED AND WHEN: Roots, in late summer or early fall.

USES: Indian women, after giving birth to a child, drank the mashed roots boiled in water. In the old South, this plant was widely used to treat constipation; to induce vomiting, and as a cure for syphilis, skin and pulmonary diseases, and liver ailments. A rubdown of boiled, mashed roots was used to treat women suffering from menstrual irregularity.

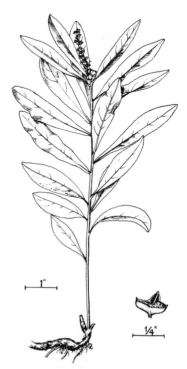

1"

1/4"

Symplocarpus foetidus (L.) Nutt.

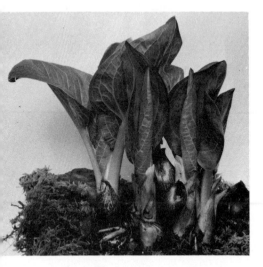

WHERE IT GROWS: Swampy and wet areas in woods, and along stream banks and springs in shaded areas. New England south to Georgia and to Tennessee, West Virginia, and Kentucky; west to Iowa, Ohio, Illinois, and Indiana.

WHAT IS HARVESTED AND WHEN: Roots and leaves, as needed.

USES: The dried ground root has been mixed with honey and taken to treat asthma and chest ailments. A salve made of the dried powdered root mixed with some carrier has been used to treat ringworm, rheumatism, and skin itching. Indians used the roots and leaves as a poultice for sores and swellings and to help draw out thorns, stickers, and splinters. The odor of the plant was sometimes inhaled to relieve headaches. The tubers have been used to treat hysteria, coughs, and epilepsy, to expel intestinal worms, and to increase menstrual flow.

OTHER COMMON NAME: pole-cat weed.

PLANT DESCRIPTION: A perennial with a distinct skunky odor. The leaves are heart-shaped, 12 to 24 inches long. The flowers, spotted and striped purple and yellow-green, appear in a spike.

Tanacetum vulgare L.

OTHER COMMON NAMES: bitter buttons, common tansy, double tansy, English cast, ginger plant, golden buttons, hindheal, parsley fern, scented fern.

PLANT DESCRIPTION: A perennial growing to 3 feet in height, characterized by a strong, aromatic odor. The leaflets are toothed; flowers, greenish and inconspicuous.

WHERE IT GROWS: Roadsides and edges of cultivated fields. Throughout the United States.

WHAT IS HARVESTED AND WHEN:
Leaves, flowering tops, and seeds, as
available.

USES: An infusion of the dried or green
leaves was used in the early 1800's to
calm nervous patients and enable them to
sleep. The bruised leaves have been used
as a poultice for bruises, sprains, and
stomachache. An oil from the plant was
used to induce abortion, often with fatal
results. The flowering tops were used to
make a tea to promote menstruation.
Indians made a steam bath with the leaves
to relieve aching feet. The dried leaves
and flowering tops have been used to
treat intestinal worms and to kill fleas,
ticks, and insects. The ground, powdered
seeds have been used as an insecticide.

240   **241**

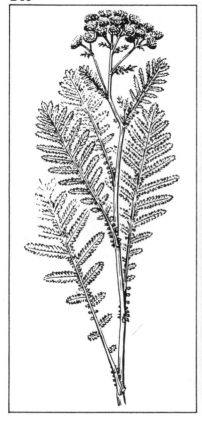

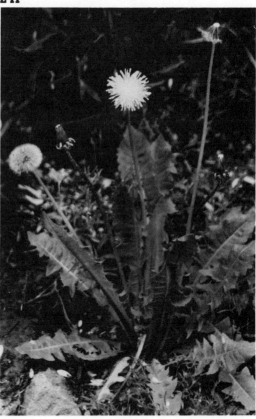

DANDELION   241

Taraxacum officinale Weber

OTHER COMMON NAMES: achicoria
amarga, blowball cankerwort, chicoria,
conseuelda, doonheadclock, fortuneteller,
Irish daisy, lion's tooth, pissabed, priest's
crown, puffball, swine snort.

PLANT DESCRIPTION: A biennial or perennial growing 2 to 12 inches tall. The deeply serrated leaves form a basal rosette in the spring. The flowers are bright yellow, maturing to gray when fruiting.

WHERE IT GROWS: Almost anywhere, in all parts of the United States, particularly on lawns.

WHAT IS HARVESTED AND WHEN: Flowers, as they appear during the growing season; roots, in late summer and early fall; green leaves, as needed.

USES: The roots have been used to increase urine flow, as a laxative and tonic, to treat liver and spleen ailments, and to stimulate the appetite. In New Mexico, a tea made of the boiled flowers has been used for heart trouble. In pioneer times, the juice of the roots was used to treat liver diseases. Indians cooked and ate the young greens in the early spring to purify the blood, and made a root tea to cure heartburn. A paste made of ground leaves and bread dough has been applied to bruises. The leaves are commonly used for salad greens, and the flowers to make a wine.

PACIFIC YEW 242

Taxus brevifolia Nutt.

OTHER COMMON NAMES: mountain mahogany, western yew, yew.

PLANT DESCRIPTION: A small evergreen tree or shrub that grows 6 to 8 feet in height. The bark is brown or dark

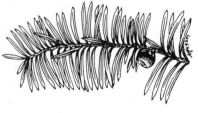

purple. The branches are spreading and almost horizontal. The needles are long and flat, tapering to a point, dark green and smooth on the upper surface. The leafstalks are almost rudimentary. The red fruits open at the top.

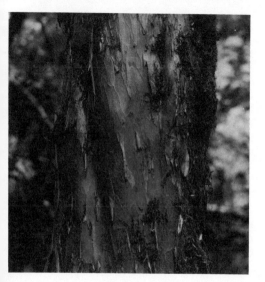

WHERE IT GROWS: In cool, damp places, such as the banks of mountain streams; in deep gorges and ravines; and in coniferous woods and bogs. Southern Alaska to Washington, Oregon, the coast of California, northern Montana, in the east, from New England south to Pennsylvania, Virginia, Kentucky, Ohio, Indiana, Illinois, Michigan, Minnesota, and Iowa.

WHAT IS HARVESTED AND WHEN:
Leaves, as needed.

USES: The leaves are supposedly useful for inducing menstruation.

VIRGINIA TEPHROSIA   243

Tephrosia virginiana (L.) Pers.

OTHER COMMON NAMES: catgut, devil's shoe strings, goat's rue, hoary pea, rabbit pea, turkey pea.

PLANT DESCRIPTION: A perennial that grows to 2 feet in height. Its erect, hairy stem is not branched and has leaves all the way to the top. The flowers occur on a terminal spike, yellow-white with purple markings. The fruits are pods, very fuzzy and 2 inches in length.

WHERE IT GROWS: Old fields, dry, sandy woods, and clearings. New England to Florida and Texas, Michigan, Wisconsin, Oklahoma, and Missouri.

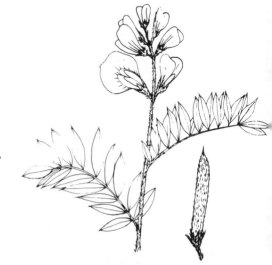

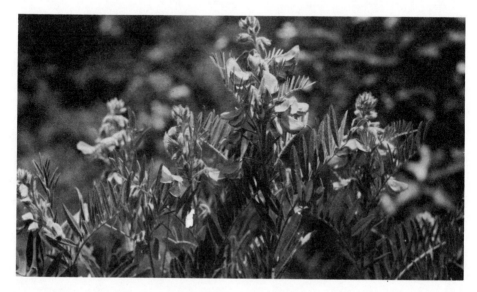

WHAT IS HARVESTED AND WHEN:
Entire plant, in full bloom; roots, in the fall.

USES: Indians used a decoction of the roots to treat intestinal worms, bladder trouble, and chronic coughing; the women used it as a shampoo to prevent falling hair. A decoction of the plant was applied by the Indians to the limbs to strengthen them for athletic participation.

Both the plant and the root have been considered helpful in treating syphilis and worms and as a tonic, stimulant, and laxative.

FENDLER MEADOWRUE   244

Thalictrum fendleri Engelm.

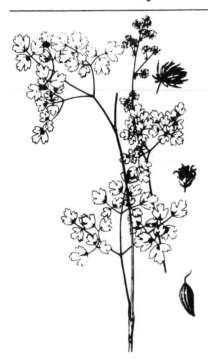

OTHER COMMON NAMES: ruda cimarron, ruda de la sierra.

PLANT DESCRIPTION: A perennial 10 to 20 inches in height. The leaflets are round to heart-shaped, three-lobed, with wavy margins. The flowers are yellow and purple.

WHERE IT GROWS: Forests, ravines and arroyos, mountains, and moist high places. Rocky Mountain area, California to Nevada, Wyoming to New Mexico, Arizona, and Colorado.

WHAT IS HARVESTED AND WHEN: Entire plant, at full bloom.

USES: In New Mexico the dried plant is rolled into a cigarette and smoked, or sprinkled on a fire, to treat headaches.

NORTHERN WHITE-CEDAR   245

Thuja occidentalis L.

OTHER COMMON NAMES: American arborvitae, arborvitae, Atlantic red cedar, cedar, eastern arborvitae, eastern white-cedar, featherleaf cedar, hack-matack, Michigan white cedar, New Brunswick cedar, swamp cedar, thuja, tree-of-life, western arborvitae, western thuja, white cedar, yellow cedar.

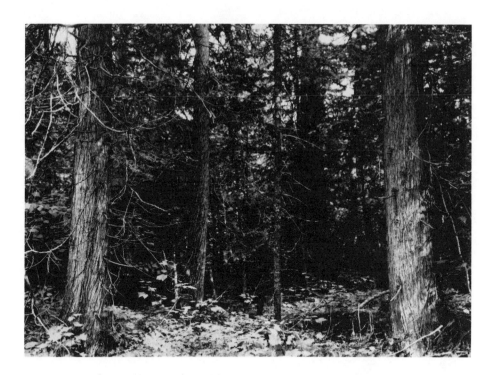

PLANT DESCRIPTION: An evergreen tree growing to 60 feet in height. The branches are horizontal, with the ends turned up. The needles are bright green above, yellow-green beneath. The cones are ½ inch long, brownish yellow. The seeds are winged.

WHERE IT GROWS: Damp and moist soils in swampy areas and on stream banks, forming forests in some places. New England south to North Carolina at higher elevations; the Appalachian region, west to Ohio, Indiana, and Illinois.

WHAT IS HARVESTED AND WHEN: Leafy young twigs, in the spring; cones, in late summer and early fall.

USES: An ointment made of fresh leaves and grease, often bear grease, was used by early settlers for treating rheumatism. A decoction of the fresh leaves was used to treat coughs, fever, and gout.

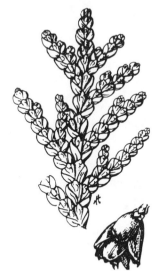

The cones were ground into a powder, mixed with milk and fern leaves, and rubbed on rheumatic joints. The leaves were also used to treat coughs, fever, scurvy, and warts, and to increase perspiration and urine flow.

ALLEGHENY FOAMFLOWER   246

Tiarella cordifolia L.

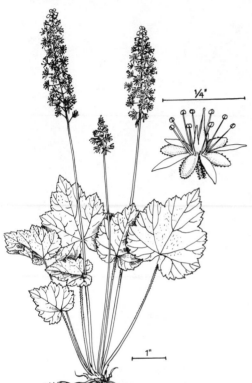

OTHER COMMON NAMES: coalwort, colwort, coolwort, false bitterwort, false miterwort, foam flower, gem fruit.

PLANT DESCRIPTION: A perennial that grows to 1 foot or more in height. The heart-shaped leaves are 4 inches across, toothed. The flowers are white to pink, on a spikelike stem.

WHERE IT GROWS: Rich woods and moist areas. New England west to Michigan and south to North Carolina, Tennessee, Kentucky, Georgia, Mississippi, and Alabama.

WHAT IS HARVESTED AND WHEN: Entire plant, during blooming period; roots, in the fall.

USES: The plant has been used in a tea to increase urine flow, help pass kidney stones, and for other urinary problems. The root has been used to increase urine flow and to loosen phlegm in the chest.

RED CLOVER   247

Trifolium pratense L.

OTHER COMMON NAMES: broad-leaved clover, cleaver grass, common clover, common red clover, cow clover, meadow clover, purple clover, sweet clover.

PLANT DESCRIPTION: A biennial or perennial legume less than 2 feet in height, with leaves consisting of three oval-shaped leaflets. The globe-shaped flowers are rose- to purple-colored.

WHERE IT GROWS: In fields and roadsides, clearings, turf, and meadows. Throughout the United States.

218

WHAT IS HARVESTED AND WHEN:
Entire plant, at full bloom.

USES: An infusion has been used to treat whooping cough and also, as a component of salves, to treat skin sores and ulcers. Indians used the plant for sore eyes and in a salve for burns. The flowers have been considered useful in treating coughs and as a sedative. In Central Europe, the plant has been used to relieve digestive distress and liver ailments, and to improve the appetite. In Ireland, during famines, the flowers have been mixed with flour as a "stretcher" in making bread.

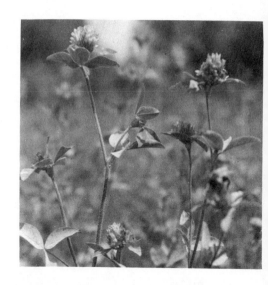

VANILLA TRILISA   248

Trilisa odoratissima (J. F. Gmel.) Cass

OTHER COMMON NAMES: deers-tongue, dogtongue, hounds-tongue, vanilla leaf, vanilla plant.

PLANT DESCRIPTION: A perennial herb 2 to 4 feet in height, with a stem growing from a cluster of leaves. The

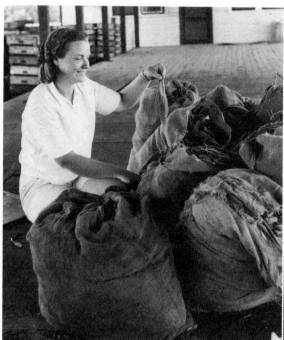

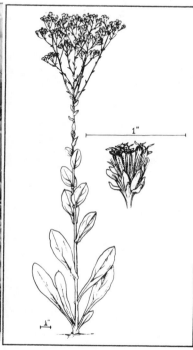

leaves are 4 to 10 inches wide, pale green. The purple flowers appear in a flat-topped terminal group.

WHERE IT GROWS: Open fields, pine barrens, and sandy woods. The Carolinas, Georgia, and Florida along the Atlantic coastal plains, and along the Gulf of Mexico to Texas.

WHAT IS HARVESTED AND WHEN: Leaves, when full size.

USES: The leaves are rich in coumarin, a vanilla-like flavoring, and are used to flavor tobacco for pipes and cigars. They have been made into a tonic to treat malaria.

PURPLE TRILLIUM 249

Trillium erectum L.

OTHER COMMON NAMES: bath flower, bathwort, bethroot, bettroot, birthroot, birthwort, bumblebee root, daffy-down-dilly, dishcloth, ground lily, ill-scented trillium, illscented wakerobin, Indian balm, Indian shamrock, lamb's quarters, nosebleed, orange blossom, purple wakerobin, rattlesnake root, red Benjamin, red trillium, squaw flower, squaw root, stinking Benjamin, three-leaved nightshade, trillium, true love, wood lily.

PLANT DESCRIPTION: A perennial that grows to 2 feet in height. It has a single stem with a whorl of three broad leaves at the top. A single brown or greenish purple flower occurs at the center of the whorl of leaves.

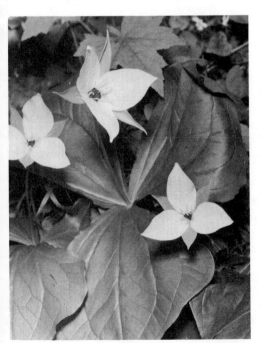

WHERE IT GROWS: Mountains and rich, moist woods. New England west to Michigan and south to West Virginia, North Carolina, Tennessee, Kentucky, and Georgia.

WHAT IS HARVESTED AND WHEN: Roots, in late summer or fall.

USES: Southeastern Indians used pieces of the root in food as an aphrodisiac. In the 1800's, chewing the root was believed to help slow down heart palpitations. The root has also been used to control hemorrhages and skin infections, and to ease the pains of childbirth.

EASTERN HEMLOCK   250

Tsuga canadensis (L.) Carr.

OTHER COMMON NAMES: Canada hemlock, hemlock, hemlock fir, hemlock spruce, hemlock spruce pine, red hemlock, spruce, spruce pine, tan-bark tree, water spruce, weeping spruce, white hemlock, Wisconsin white hemlock pine.

PLANT DESCRIPTION: An evergreen tree growing to 75 feet in height. The needles are 1/3 to 2/3 inch long, flattened, tapering to a point, bright green

woods, moist soils, the banks of river gorges, and the slopes of rocky ridges. New York, Pennsylvania, Minnesota, Wisconsin, Michigan, and Indiana, south to Maryland, and along the Appalachian Mountains to Georgia and Alabama.

WHAT IS HARVESTED AND WHEN: Bark, as needed; resin (collected by cutting the trunk of the tree), usually during the growing season; needles, as needed.

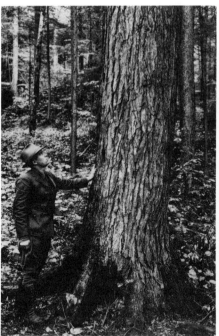 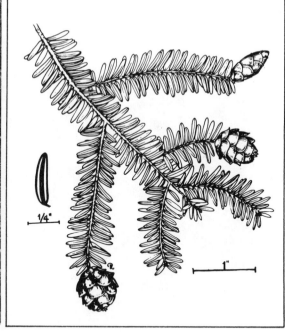

above and light green, with two white streaks, below. The cones are small, 1/2 to 3/4 inch long. The bark is deeply furrowed and dark reddish brown.

WHERE IT GROWS: A very wide range of habitats: upland mountainous rocky

USES: Indians boiled the inner bark, pounded it, and applied it to swellings and sores. They made a tea from the needles and used it for making a sick person sweat, and to treat colds, coughs, and flu. The resin has been used to form skin blisters.

Typha latifolia L.

OTHER COMMON NAMES: broad-leaved cattail, bulrush, cat tail, flag.

PLANT DESCRIPTION: A perennial marsh plant growing to 6 feet in height. The leaves are long and linear, arising from the base of the stem and growing to 4 feet in length. The flowers are clustered in a dense spike.

WHERE IT GROWS: Marshes or shallow water, irrigation ditches, swampy areas, and stagnant pools. Throughout the United States.

WHAT IS HARVESTED AND WHEN: Roots, as needed; seeds, in the fall; the down, at flowering.

USES: In colonial times, poorer settlers in Virginia ate the part of stem at the very base, near the origin of the roots, and roasted the seeds to eat as a vegetable. The chopped root was applied to the skin for minor wounds and burns; it was also used to treat diarrhea, gonorrhea, and worms. The down was used as a treatment for burns.

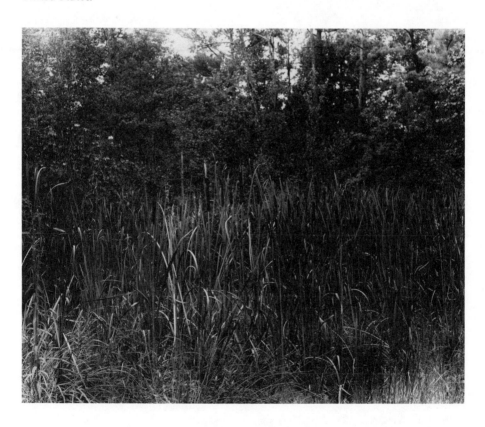

AMERICAN ELM   252

Ulmus americana L.

OTHER COMMON NAMES: soft elm, water elm, white elm.

PLANT DESCRIPTION: A spreading tree that grows to 120 feet in height. The bark is gray and flaky. The leaves are 3

shade tree. Widely distributed in the northeastern states, South Dakota, Montana, Wyoming, Kansas, Oklahoma, Texas, and as far south as Florida.

WHAT IS HARVESTED AND WHEN:

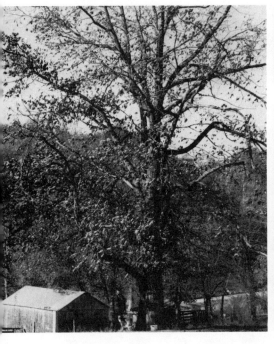

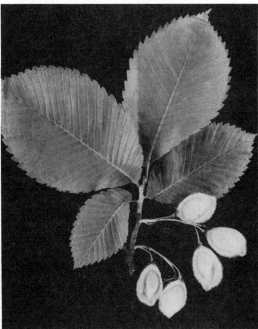

to 6 inches long, roughened above, fuzzy below. The flowers are borne in hanging clusters. The fruit is flattened, round, about ½ inch long, with hairy, notched margins.

WHERE IT GROWS: Fertile soils in forests and river bottoms; planted as a

Bark, as needed.

USES: The ground bark has been made into a poultice for skin inflammations and abrasions. An infusion of the bark has been used to treat dysentery and kidney ailments. The inner bark has been used as a tonic and to increase urine flow.

Ulmus rubra Muhl.

OTHER COMMON NAMES: American tree, elm, gray elm, Indian elm, moose elm, red elm, rock elm, soft elm, sweet elm, tawny elm.

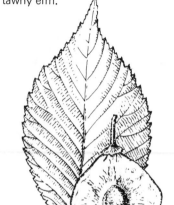

WHERE IT GROWS: Widely distributed in moist woods, stream banks, bottomlands, hillsides, and on poor and dry sites. Maine and New Hampshire to Michigan, Wisconsin, Minnesota, North Dakota, Oklahoma, Texas, Georgia, Florida, Alabama, Mississippi, Virginia, Kentucky, and West Virginia.

WHAT IS HARVESTED AND WHEN: Inner bark, in spring or fall; roots, at any time.

USES: In Appalachia, a tea made from the bark is used as a laxative. After the inner bark has been soaked in warm water, it produces a mucilage that has been used to soften the skin and protect it from chapping, to hasten the healing of

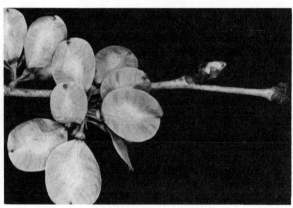

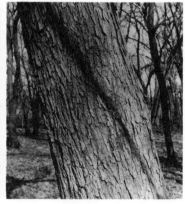

PLANT DESCRIPTION: A tree that grows to 75 feet in height. The leaves are dark green, 6 to 7 inches long, 2 to 3 inches wide, rough above and fuzzy below, almost oval in shape. The buds at the ends of the branches often have orange tips. The inner bark is sticky and has an aromatic flavor.

skin wounds, and as a laxative. Bark poultices have been applied to burns. Indians used the bark, beaten to a pulp, to treat gunshot wounds and help remove bullets. They also used it to treat fever, diarrhea, and respiratory infections, and made a tea from boiled roots to assist women in childbirth.

CALIFORNIA LAUREL   254

Umbellularia californica Nutt.

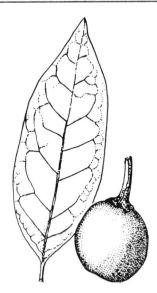

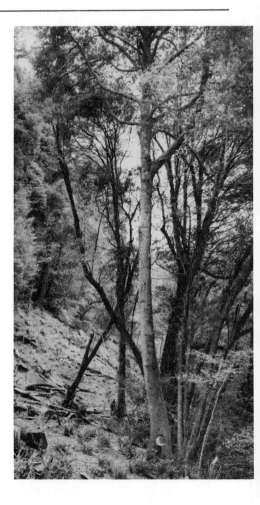

OTHER COMMON NAMES: bay, bay laurel, bay tree, black myrtle, cajeput, California baytree, California olive, California sassafras, creodaphne, laurel, mountain laurel, myrtle, Oregon myrtle, oreodaphne, pepperwood, spice tree, white myrtle, yellow myrtle.

PLANT DESCRIPTION: An evergreen tree growing to a height of 50 to 75 feet. The pungently aromatic leaves are 3 to 5 inches long, shiny and leathery. The flowers grow in clusters 1½ to 2 inches across, yellowish green, followed by fruits 1 inch long, purplish to yellow-green.

WHERE IT GROWS: Alluvial deposits and areas of sedimentary rock. Oregon to California.

WHAT IS HARVESTED AND WHEN: Leaves, as needed.

USES: The pioneers tied the leaves to the forehead or put a leaf in a nostril as a treatment for headache. For chronic stomach trouble, the leaves were bound around the body. A tea made of leaves has been used to treat headaches and stomach troubles. The leaves were also put into hot baths to treat rheumatism. California Indians used them to repel fleas and other biting insects.

SPARKLEBERRY 255

Vaccinium arboreum Marsh.

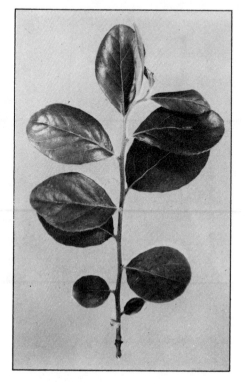

OTHER COMMON NAMES: farkleberry, gooseberry, huckleberry, whortleberry.

PLANT DESCRIPTION: A shrub or tree growing to 25 feet in height. The leaves are shiny, thick, and leathery. The flowers are white, the berries black.

WHERE IT GROWS: Woods, clearings, sandy and dry woods. Virginia, Georgia, Florida, Mississippi, Appalachian region, Indiana, Illinois, Missouri, Texas, and Oklahoma.

WHAT IS HARVESTED AND WHEN: Leaves, when mature; root bark, in spring or fall; fruits, in summer and fall.

USES: The leaves and the bark of the root have been used in decoctions to treat sore throat and diarrhea. The fruit has been used to make a drink for treating chronic dysentery.

FALSE HELLEBORE 256

Veratrum californicum E. Durand.

OTHER COMMON NAMES: corn-lily, false white hellebore, skunk-cabbage, tailed-false hellebore.

PLANT DESCRIPTION: A perennial growing to 2 feet in height. The leaves are large, coarse, parallel-veined, with fine hairs. The flowers are greenish or cream-colored.

WHERE IT GROWS: Bogs and wet meadows, stream banks, mountain meadows, and wet woods. Montana to Washington, south to New Mexico, Arizona, Colorado, and California.

WHAT IS HARVESTED AND WHEN: Roots, as needed.

USES: A decoction of the root has been used by Indians as a birth-control measure; taken daily for three weeks, it was be-lieved to prevent conception. The water in which the roots were boiled was con-sidered effective in killing head lice.

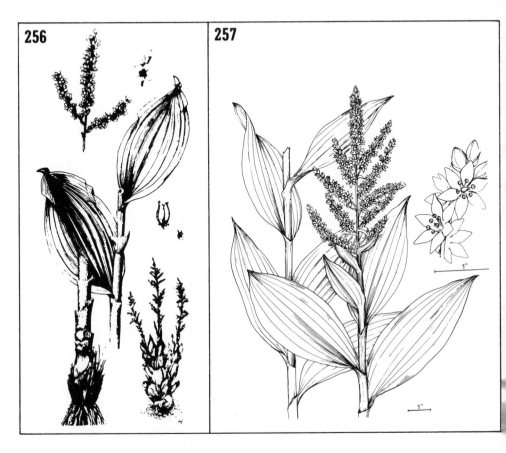

WHITE HELLEBORE   257

Veratrum viride Ait.

OTHER COMMON NAMES: American falsehellebore, American hellebore, American white hellebore, bear-corn, big-bane, common swamp hellebore, devil's-bite, false hellebore, green false hellebore, green hellebore, Indian itch-weed, pokeweed, swamp hellebore.

PLANT DESCRIPTION: An erect pe-rennial 2 to 8 feet in height. The stems are leafy, unbranched, and arise from · short, thick rootstocks. The leaves are alternate, ovate to elliptical, with parallel veining. The flowers are greenish white to purple, inconspicuous, and borne in pyramidal clusters 2 feet long.

WHERE IT GROWS: Wet woods, swamps , stream banks, and low mead-ows. In the East, New York and New

England, south to Georgia, North Carolina, Tennessee, and West Virginia, and west to Wisconsin; in the Northwest, the Cascade Mountains and Oregon.

WHAT IS HARVESTED AND WHEN:
Roots and rhizomes, in the fall after the leaves have died.

USES: Indians rubbed a wound with wildcat or raccoon grease, then covered the area with powdered root. A dangerous treatment for toothache (the plant is extremely poisonous) was to put the root powder into the tooth. Colonists used the roots, sliced thin and boiled in vinegar, as an external application to treat "shingles" or herpes. They also boiled the root, dipped a comb in the brew, and combed their own and their children's hair to kill lice. The dried roots and rhizomes have been used in heart cases, to reduce high blood pressure, and in the treatment of asthma, indigestion, rheumatism, and gout.

COMMON MULLEIN   258

Verbascum thapsus L.

OTHER COMMON NAMES: Aaron's rod, Adam's flannel, blanket leaf, bullock's lungwort, candlewick, cow's lungwort, feltwort, flannel leaf, flannel mullein, flannel plant, great mullein, hare's beard, hedge taper, ice leaf, Indian tobacco, Jacob's staff, Jupiter's staff, lady's foxglove, mullein, mullein dock, old man's flannel, Peter's staff, shepherd's club, torch-wort, velvet dock, velvet plant.

PLANT DESCRIPTION: The hairy rosette of lance-shaped and oblong leaves at the base, with a diameter up to 2 feet, gives rise to a seed stalk that grows to a height of 7 feet. The yellow flowers are arranged densely along a clublike spike.

WHERE IT GROWS: Along railroad tracks; in dry fields and meadows, pastures, rocky or gravelly banks, overgrazed or burned areas; around settlements; and in open forests. It apparently occurs in all parts of the United States from Maine to Florida, in New Mexico and Arizona, Colorado to California.

WHAT IS HARVESTED AND WHEN:
Leaves, when large enough and through maturity; roots, in the fall; flowers, as they appear in spring.

USES: In Appalachia, a tea made from the leaves is used to treat colds; in other places, the leaf tea is a treatment for dysentery. A number of Indian tribes smoked the leaves for asthma and sore throat; others boiled the roots, sweetened them, and fed the mixture to children with croup. Some early settlers tied the hairy leaves around their feet and arms to treat malaria. Mullein leaves and flowers have been considered soothing for mucous membranes. The leaves have been used to soften the skin and protect it. The flowers have been used to treat diseases of the chest and

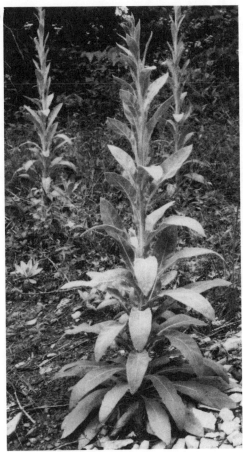
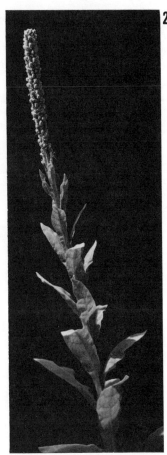

lungs. The flowers contain an oil that has been used for earache. The leaves have been used as local applications for hemorrhoids, sunburn, and inflammations.

BLUE VERVAIN   259

Verbena hastata L.

OTHER COMMON NAMES: blue verbena, ironweed, simpler's joy, tall wild verbena, verbain, wild hyssop.

PLANT DESCRIPTION: A perennial that grows to 4 feet in height. The leaves have serrated edges and are three-lobed, with two sharp lobes arising from the base. The blue and blue-violet flowers are produced on numerous terminal spikes.

WHERE IT GROWS: Very widely adapted to many habitats, it is found along irrigation ditches and shores; in damp thickets, moist fields, meadows, waste places; on riverbottoms and prairies. New England and Long Island south

229

to Virginia, North Carolina, Georgia, Florida, Tennessee, West Virginia, Kentucky, Missouri, Texas, New Mexico, Arizona, Colorado, and California.

WHAT IS HARVESTED AND WHEN:
Roots, at any time; above-ground parts, at full bloom.

USES: Indians used a tea made of boiled leaves for stomachache, and a tea made of the roots to clear up cloudy urine. During the American Revolution, doctors used verbena to induce vomiting and to clear the respiratory tracts of mucus. It has also been used to increase perspiration in persons with a low fever and a cold.

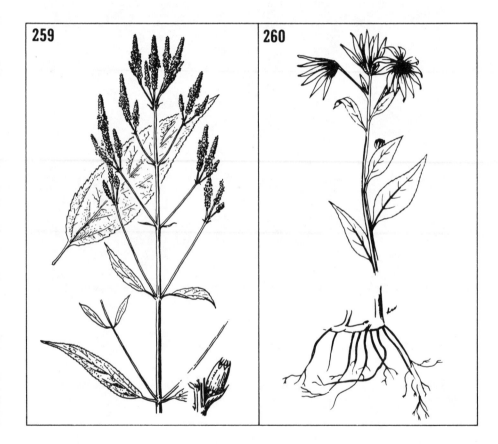

259

260

CROWNBEARD   260

Verbesina helianthoides Michx.

OTHER COMMON NAMES: diabetes weed, gravelweed, sunflower crownbeard.

PLANT DESCRIPTION: A perennial growing to 3 feet in height, with coarse hairs on the stem. The leaves are rough above and hairy beneath. The flowers are yellow.

WHERE IT GROWS: Thickets and prairies, open woods. Ohio and Missouri, Texas to Georgia.

WHAT IS HARVESTED AND WHEN: Roots, in the fall from plants older than one year; entire plant, at full bloom.

USES: A root infusion has been used to treat water retention and bladder inflammation, and to purify the blood. A tea made from the plant has been used for stomach distress. In New Mexico, a close relative of this plant has been mixed with tobacco and made into a poultice for treating hemorrhoids.

CULVER'S PHYSIC   261

Veronicastrum virginicum (L.) Farw.

OTHER COMMON NAMES: Beaumont root, black-root, bowman's root, Culver's root, physic root, tall speedwell, whorlywort.

PLANT DESCRIPTION: An erect, unbranched perennial that grows to 6 feet in height. The leaves are narrow and lance-shaped, growing in whorls of three or more at the stem joints. The flowers are white to blue, and occur in dense spikes at the top of the plant.

WHERE IT GROWS: In a range of habitats from dry or moist uplands to rich, moist woods and thickets, moist meadows, and prairies. Massachusetts and Vermont south to North Carolina, South Carolina, Florida, Mississippi, Louisiana, and Texas.

WHAT IS HARVESTED AND WHEN: Rhizomes and roots, as needed, but preferably during the growing season and from plants at least two years old.

USES: The dried tubers are a mild laxa-

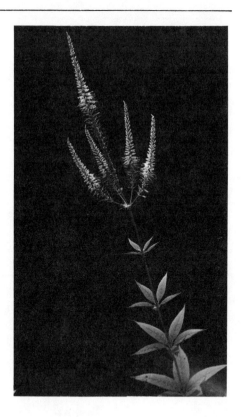

tive. Indians used them for this purpose and to induce vomiting.

POSSUMHAW VIBURNUM 262

Viburnum nudum L.

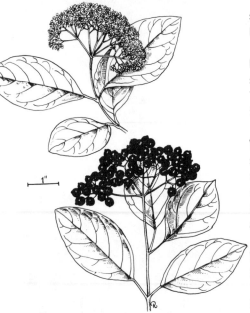

OTHER COMMON NAMES: larger withe-root, possumhaw, shawnee haw, shonny haw, smooth withe-rod, swamp haw, white rod.

PLANT DESCRIPTION: A perennial shrub that grows to 20 feet in height. The leaves are up to 5 inches long. The flowers are white or sometimes pink.

WHERE IT GROWS: Rich, moist hill-sides; low, moist areas near streams; moist woods; and open glades. Connecticut to Florida along the coast and piedmont, Louisiana to Arkansas and Texas, and inland to Tennessee and Kentucky.

WHAT IS HARVESTED AND WHEN: Bark of root or stem, as needed.

USES: The bark has been used to treat malaria and uterine disorders, as a tonic, and to increase urine flow.

HIGHBUSH CRANBERRY 263

Viburnum opulus L.

OTHER COMMON NAMES: cramp bark, cranberry tree, European cranberry bush, guelder-rose, high cranberry.

PLANT DESCRIPTION: A shrub growing to 12 feet in height, with smooth, light-gray branches. The leaves are 2 to 4 inches long, three-lobed, toothed, hairy beneath. The flowers are white; the fruit scarlet, ½ inch in diameter.

WHERE IT GROWS: Wet places, along stream banks, near swamps, and low, poorly drained areas. Throughout the United States.

WHAT IS HARVESTED AND WHEN: Bark, as needed; berries, in late summer when ripe.

USES: The bark has been used to treat uterine infections and septic poisoning during childbirth. Indians used it to increase urine flow. The berries are a good source of vitamin C and have been used to treat scurvy.

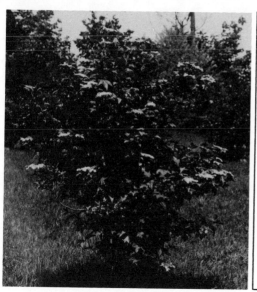

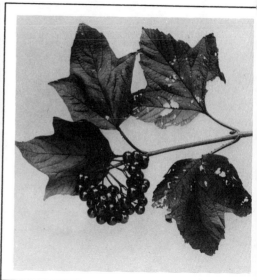

BLACK HAW 264

Viburnum prunifolium L.

OTHER COMMON NAMES: blackhaw viburnum, cramp bark, sheepberry, shonny, sloe, sloe-leaved viburnum, stagbush, sweethaw.

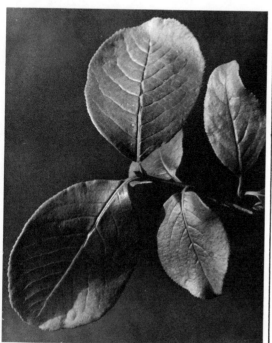

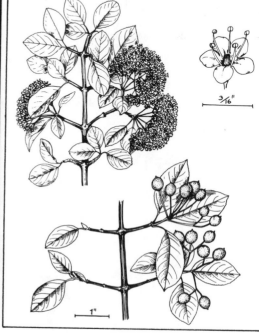

PLANT DESCRIPTION: A perennial shrub or small tree, 10 to 20 feet in height, with spreading branches. The dull-colored leaves are ovate, opposite, and stemmed, with finely serrated margins. The plant produces white flowers and dullish black, oval fruits.

WHERE IT GROWS: Dry, rocky hillsides, fence rows, roadsides, thickets, borders of woods, and shores, on dry or moist soils. Florida to Texas, north to New York, Connecticut, Ohio, Michigan, Illinois, Iowa, and Kansas.

WHAT IS HARVESTED AND WHEN: Stems and rootbark, in the fall; twigs, during the growing season.

USES: In Appalachia, a tea made of the root bark is used as a tonic. A decoction of the bark has been used to treat uterine hemorrhage, and a decoction of twigs to treat diarrhea, uterine pains, and general spasms.

BROAD BEAN   265

Vicia faba L.

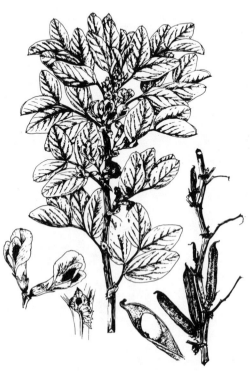

OTHER COMMON NAMES: English bean, horse bean; mazagon, windsor.

PLANT DESCRIPTION: A vigorously growing, hardy, erect annual, 2 to 6 feet in height, very heavily leaved. The leaflets are found in one to three pairs, alternate, 2 to 4 inches long. The terminal leaflet is usually a tendril. The flowers are 1 to 1½ inches long, white with purple touches. The beans are flat, 1 to 1½ inches long, of various colors.

WHERE IT GROWS: The plant is cultivated and grown all over the United States.

WHAT IS HARVESTED AND WHEN: Pod (beans), when ripe in late summer.

USES: This is one of the most ancient of our cultivated edible plants. It has been found in Bronze Age deposits in Switzerland, and was grown by the Hebrews,

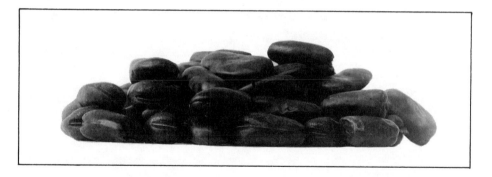

Greeks, Egyptians, and Romans. The ground dried beans have been used to treat mouth sores. In New Mexico, a paste made of ground beans and hot water is applied to the chest and back as a treatment for pneumonia.

CANADA VIOLET 266

Viola canadensis L.

OTHER COMMON NAME: tall white violet.

PLANT DESCRIPTION: A violet with a white flower, sometimes touched with violet color. It reaches a height of 18 inches, and the leaves have deep indentations.

WHERE IT GROWS: In woods and forests. Eastern United States as far south as South Carolina and Alabama, and west to Utah, Colorado, and South Dakota.

WHAT IS HARVESTED AND WHEN: Entire plant and roots, as needed.

USES: The tops and the roots have been used to induce vomiting and to serve as laxatives. A poultice of the plant parts has been applied to skin abrasions.

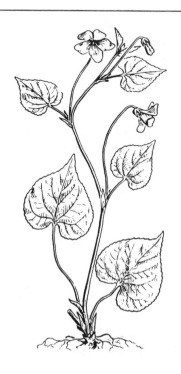

BIRDSFOOT VIOLET   267

Viola pedata L.

OTHER COMMON NAMES: crowfoot violet, garden violet, pansy, pansy violet, parsley violet, sweet violet, violet.

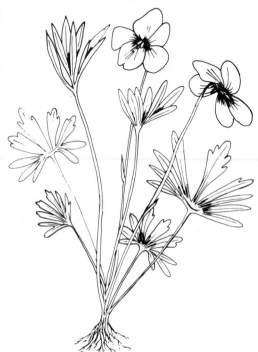

PLANT DESCRIPTION: A low-growing perennial with leaves divided into three lobes. The dark violet flowers are borne on 2-to-6-inch-long stems, and are ¾ to 1½ inches across. The plant may easily be confused with its many related species.

WHERE IT GROWS: A wide range of soils in sunny areas. Eastern states and the Appalachian area to Louisiana, Missouri, and Florida; some varieties as far west as Minnesota and Kansas.

WHAT IS HARVESTED AND WHEN: Roots, in late summer or early fall; aboveground plant, when in bloom.

USES: The plant parts and roots have been used as a mild laxative and to induce vomiting. A decoction of the aboveground parts has been used to loosen phlegm in the chest, and for other pulmonary problems.

COMMON COCKLEBUR   268

Xanthium strumarium L.

OTHER COMMON NAMES: broad cocklebur, burweed, sea burdock.

PLANT DESCRIPTION: An annual growing to 5 feet in height. The leaves and stems are hairy; the flowers greenish and inconspicuous; the burs yellow green and hairy, less than 1 inch long.

WHERE IT GROWS: Dry areas, old

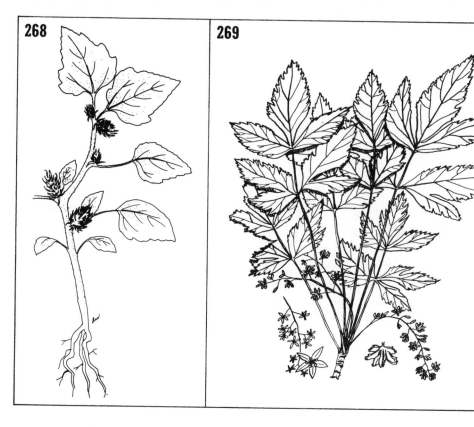

fields, roadsides, stream banks, and beaches. Throughout the United States.

WHAT IS HARVESTED AND WHEN: Leaves, when mature.

USES: The leaves have been used to treat tuberculosis of the neck glands, "shingles" (herpes), and skin and bladder infections, and also to stop the bleeding of skin cuts and abrasions.

YELLOW ROOT   269

Xanthorhiza simplicissima Marsh.

OTHER COMMON NAME: shrub yellowroot.

PLANT DESCRIPTION: A perennial low shrub that grows to 1½ feet in height. It bears a cluster of compound leaves, each with five lance-shaped to oval, toothed, incised, or parted leaflets. The flowers are small, purplish brown, borne on thin spikes. The wood is bright yellow.

WHERE IT GROWS: Chiefly in mountain areas, preferring damp woods, stream banks, and thickets. New York and Pennsylvania to Kentucky and West Virginia, South Carolina, Florida, and Alabama.

WHAT IS HARVESTED AND WHEN: Roots, at any time.

USES: The root has been used as a tonic and in the treatment of dyspepsia. People in Appalachia drink tea made from the root for throat and stomach disorders. Indians made such a decoction to help a mother in childbirth. Sometimes they chewed fresh or dried roots to relieve stomach distress, and used the boiled roots to treat jaundice, sore mouth, and colds.

PRICKLYASH   270

Xanthoxylum americanum Mill.

OTHER COMMON NAMES: American pricklyash, common pricklyash, northern pricklyash, pellitory bark, toothache bush, toothache tree, yellow wood.

PLANT DESCRIPTION: A shrub or small tree growing from 5 to 10 feet in height. The leaves are alternate and compound, with five to eleven leaflets. The stems and petioles are often prickly. The greenish white flowers are small and inconspicuous. The fruit is reddish, globe-shaped, and aromatic.

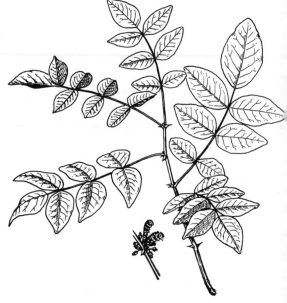

WHERE IT GROWS: Riverbanks and rich, moist woods. New England south to Alabama, Mississippi, Florida, Georgia, Kentucky, West Virginia, and Virginia, and west to North Dakota and Oklahoma.

WHAT IS HARVESTED AND WHEN: Fruit, when ripe; bark of stem and root, in spring and fall.

USES: Indians chewed the bark for toothache, used a decoction of the bark to treat colic, rheumatism, and gonorrhea, and made it into a poultice, with bear grease, to treat sores and ulcers. They applied the bark to infected wounds to draw out the pus. An ounce of bark boiled in a quart of water, drunk at the rate of a pint a day, was a treatment for rheumatism. The scraped root has been used to treat ulcers. The seeds were a remedy for toothache; the berries were used in cough syrup to induce the coughing up of phlegm. The ripe berries cooked in hot water produced a spray for treating mouth sores.

Xanthoxylum clava-herculis L.

OTHER COMMON NAMES: Hercules club, pillenterry, prickly-ash, sea ash, shrubby pricklyash, southern pricklyash, sting-a-tongue, toothache tree, wait-a-bit,, wild orange.

PLANT DESCRIPTION: A shrub or small tree 5 to 10 feet in height. The leaves are alternate, compound, with five to eleven leaflets. The stems and petioles are often prickly. The flowers are greenish white, small and inconspicuous. The fruit is a reddish globular to elliptic aromatic capsule, with prickles.

WHERE IT GROWS: Sand hills, thickets, dry woods, coastal areas, riverbanks, and sand dunes. Southern Virginia, Kentucky, and West Virginia to Florida, westward through the Gulf states to Louisiana, Texas, Arkansas, and Oklahoma.

WHAT IS HARVESTED AND WHEN: Bark, in spring and fall; berries, in early fall; roots, as needed; inner bark, during the growing season; wood, as needed.

USES: Indians used this plant for an amazing range of ailments. A decoction of the bark was used for gonorrhea; the wood for toothache; and a decoction of the boiled roots to increase perspiration.

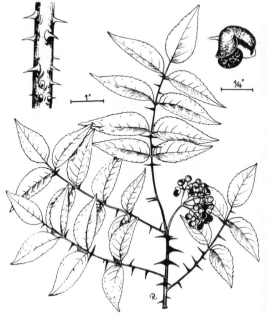

Both Indians and early settlers mixed the inner bark with bear grease and applied it as a poultice to treat ulcers. Ripe berries were thrown in hot water to make a spray used in the mouth and blown on the chest and throat for chest ailments. The bark was also used for inflammations of the throat. The inner bark, boiled in water, produced a lotion used to treat various itches. The berries have been considered tonic, stimulant, anti-rheumatic, and effective in relieving gas, colic, and muscle spasms.

Yucca brevifolia Engelm.

PLANT DESCRIPTION: A tree growing to 35 feet in height. The leaves are 4 to 6 inches long. The fruit is spongy and dry; the capsule, 2 to 4 inches long.

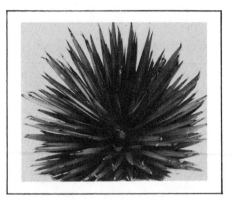

WHERE IT GROWS: Desert and semi-desert arid areas. Mohave Desert of California to Arizona, Utah, and Nevada.

WHAT IS HARVESTED AND WHEN: Roots, as needed; fruit, as mature.

USES: The crushed roots are boiled in water and the tea drunk as a treatment for gonorrhea. The fruit has been used in some Indian ceremonies to induce vomiting.

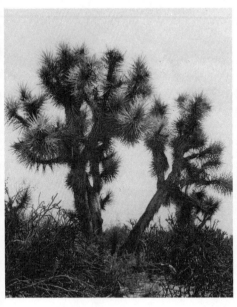
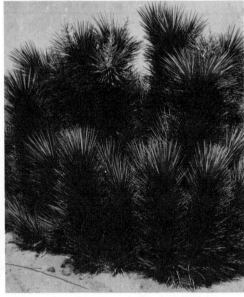

APPENDIX I

Sources of Botanical Supplies

Names	Addresses

SELLERS OF DRUG PLANT SEEDS AND PROPAGATING MATERIALS

Names	Addresses
Gardens of the Blue Ridge	Ashford, North Carolina 28603
Herbst Brothers	100 North Main St., Brewster, New York 10509
Hilltop Herb Farm	Box 366, Cleveland, Texas 77327
Indiana Botanic Gardens	P.O. Box 5, Hammond, Indiana 26325
Nichols Garden Nursery	1190 North Pacific Highway, Albany, Oregon 97321.
Harry E. Saier	Dimondale, Michigan 48821

DEALERS IN BOTANICALS AND BOTANICAL PRODUCTS

Names	Addresses
Blue Ridge Drug Company	P.O. Box 234, West Jefferson, North Carolina 28694
Boericke & Tafel	1011 Arch Street, Philadelphia, Pennsylvania 19107
Coeburn Produce Company	Second and Grand Streets, Coburn, Virginia 24230
C. R. Graybeal	Roan Mountain, Tennessee 37687
Greer & Greer	Box 307, Princeton, West Virginia 24740
Greer Drug & Chemical Company	P.O. Box 800, Lenoir, North Carolina 28645
Hathaway Allied Products	2024 Westgate Avenue, Los Angeles, California 90025
Old Fashioned Herb Company	581 North Lake Avenue, Los Angeles, California 90025
S. B. Penick & Company	100 Church Street, New York, New York 10007
Smoky Mountain Drug Company	935 Shelby Street, Box 2, Bristol, Tennessee 37620
Standard Homeopathic Pharmacy	436 West Eighth Street, Los Angeles, California 90014
F. C. Taylor Fur Company	227 East Market Street, Louisville, Kentucky 40202
Wilcox Drug Company	P.O. Box 391, Boone, North Carolina 28697
Wilcox Drug Company, Inc.	Box 470, Pikeville, Kentucky 41501

APPENDIX 2

Meanings of Plant Names

Acutiloba. Having sharp lobes.
Alba. White.
Albidum. Whitish.
Ambrosioides. Fragrant, like ambrosia.
Americanus. American.
Androsaemifolium. Having leaves like those of Androsaemum.
Aparine. Bedstraw.
Arborescens. Treelike.
Atropurpurea. Very dark purple.
Aureus. Gold.

Balsamifera. Producing balsam.
Benedictus. Blessed.
Benzoin. A plant of the laurel family.
Biflorum. Having two flowers.

Calamus. Reed.
Canadense. Of Canada.
Capillus veneris. Hairlike.
Cardiaca. Heartlike.
Carolinense. Of Carolina.
Cataria. Catnip.
Cerifera. Wax-producing.
Cinerea. Grayish.
Clava-Herculis. Hercules club.
Communis. In groups.
Cordifolia. Heart-shaped.
Crispus. Waved and twisted.

Didyma. In pairs.
Diphylla. Two-leaved.

Erectum. Erect.
Farinosa. Covered with whitish mealy powder.
Frondosa. Full of leaves.

Glabra. Smooth.
Hastata. Having triangular halberd-shaped lobes.

Hippocastanum. Horse-chestnut.
Hybridus. Mixed or impure.
Hydropiper. Water pepper.
Hyemale. Of the winter evergreen.

Incarnata. Flesh-colored.
Inflata. Expanded.

Lappa. Bur-like.
Lateriflora. Having flowers on the side.
Lenta. Pliant, tough.
Luteum. Yellow.

Maculata. Spotted.
Marilandica. Of Maryland.
Media. Middle.
Millefolium. Very many-leaved.
Minus. Lesser or smaller.

Nigra. Black.
Nudicaulis. Naked-stemmed.
Nudum. Bare.

Odoratissima. Very fragrant.
Officinale. Used medically.

Palustris. Of swamps.
Parviflorum. Small-flowered.
Pedatum. Like a bird's foot.
Peltatum. Shield-shaped.
Peregrina. Traveling from a strange country.
Perfoliatum. Having pierced leaves.
Piperita. Peppery.
Pratense. Of meadows.
Procumbens. Flat, prostrate.
Prunifolium. Plumlike leaves.
Pulegioides. Like pennyroyal.

Quinquefolium. Five-leaved.

Racemosa. Full of clusters.
Repens. Creeping.
Rubra. Red.

Scariola. Papery, scaly.
Sempervirens. Evergreen.
Serotina. Late-flowering.
Serpentaria. Snake bite cure.
Serrulata. Finely serrated.
Simplicissima. Undivided.
Spicata. Bearing a spike.
Stramonium. Swelling.
Strobus. Overlapping scales; cone.
Styraciflua. Flowering gum.

Sylvatica. Of the forest, wild.
Syriaca. Of Syria.

Thalictroides. Like meadow rue.
Thapsus. Of ancient Thapsus.
Tinctoria. Of dyes.
Triphyllum. Three-leaved.
Tuberosa. Having tubers.

Umbellata. Having flowers arranged
in umbels.

Villosa. Shaggy, hairy.
Viride. Green.
Vulgare. Common.

Illustration Credits

Smithsonian Institution, National Anthropological Archives, Washington, D.C.
Fig. 1, No. 2189; Fig. 2, No. 1641; Fig. 4, No. 1186-B-10; Fig. 5, No. 1425; Fig. 6, No. 1008; Fig. 8, No. 1459A; Fig. 9, No. 1455A; Fig. 10, No. 1456D.

New York Botanical Garden
25; 57; 70; 71; 82; 108; 129; 132; 135; 173; 179; 218; 230; 239; 265 (photo).

United States Department of Agriculture
13; 15; 18; 21 (leaves and flowers); 22; 24; 26 (leaves); 29; 38; 47; 48; 58; 63; 78 (leaves); 83; 85; 88; 89; 90; 93; 103; 109; 126; 149 (sketch); 150; 153; 154; 156; 163; 164 (sketch); 168; 170; 174; 178; 181; 186 (greens); 183; 187 (tree); 189; 193; 205; 210 (sketch); 213 (sketch); 223 (sketch); 241; 243 (sketch); 252; 254 (sketch); 265 (sketch, courtesy Mrs. R. O. Hughes); 267; 268.

Field Museum of Natural History, Chicago
27; 34 (plant); 37 (photo); 149 (photo); 215.

Dr. James Hardin, Botany Department, North Carolina State University, Raleigh, N.C.
23; 32; 61 (lower left photo); 91; 115 (photo); 121; 128; 134; 148; 164 (photo); 186 (fruit); 214.

Great Smoky Mountains National Park, Gatlinburg, Tennessee
26 (tree); 30; 42; 60; 65 (photo); 86; 169; 213 (photo); 224; 237; 243 (photo); 247; 249

University of Mississippi, School of Pharmacy, Department of Pharmacognosy
54 (photo).

University of Kentucky, Lexington
44.

Kentucky Department of Highways
34 (lower photo).

University of California at Davis, Department of Agronomy
56.

Louisville Courier Journal
186 (canned greens).

Soil Conservation Service United States Department of Agriculture
78 (fruit).

United States Forest Service
3; 7; 11; 12; 14; 16; 17; 19; 20; 21 (bark and fruit); 31; 33; 35; 36; 37 (sketch); 39; 41; 45; 49; 51; 52; 59; 61 (sketch); 64; 65 (sketch); 66; 68; 69; 73; 74; 77; 79; 80; 84; 92; 96; 98; 100; 101; 102; 104; 106; 107; 110; 111; 113; 114; 115 (sketch); 117; 119; 122; 127; 133; 138; 139; 140; 142; 143; 144; 145; 146; 151; 152; 155; 158; 159; 160; 165; 172; 175;

177; 180; 182; 184; 185; 186 (plants); 187 (bark and leaves); 188; 190; 191; 192; 194; 195; 196; 197; 198; 199; 200; 201 (photo); 202; 203; 204; 206; 207; 208; 209; 210 (photo); 211; 212; 219; 220; 222; 223 (photo); 228; 229; 231; 232; 233; 234; 236; 238; 242; 244; 245; 246; 248 (sketch); 250; 253; 254 (photo); 255; 256; 257; 258; 260; 261; 262; 264; 271; 272.

University of Arizona

(Kittie F. Parker. 1958. **Arizona Ranch, Farm and Garden Weeds.** Agricultural Extension Service Bull. 265.) 87; 99; 112; 125; 130; 147; 161; 201 (sketch).

Colorado State University

(B. L. Thornton and L. W. Durrell. **Weeds of Colorado.** Col Exp. Sta. Bull. 466,
Colo. State College, Ft. Collins. 125 pp., illus.) 28; 43; 55; 75; 76; 95; 116; 123; 124; 217; 221; 225.

Texas Research Foundation

(C. L. Lundell & collaborators. 1962. **Flora of Texas.** Vol. 2, Texas Research Foundation, Renner. 417 pp., illus.) 97; 105; 62.

University of West Virginia

(P. D. Strausbaugh, and Earl L. Core. **Flora of West Virginia,** Vols. 1, 2, 3, 4, West Virginia University Bulletins 52(12), 53(12), 58(12), 65(3), and Introductory Section 65(3)) 32 (sketch); 40; 46; 50; 53; 54 (sketch); 67; 72; 81; 94; 120; 131; 136; 137; 141; 157; 166; 167; 176; 226; 235; 240; 259; 266; 269; 270.

INDEX OF PLANT NAMES

245

246

INDEX OF AILMENTS

WARNING: This list is a historical compilation and not meant to be used for treating any of the ailments given. Wild plants are enormously variable in their constituents in terms of percentages and occurrences, and to use them involves risks.

A

abortion
Acorus calamus
Chrysanthemum parthenium
Juniperus virginiana
Nasturtium officinale
Ruta graveolens
Tanacetum vulgare

abscess
Eucalyptus globulus

aches
Helianthus annuus
Tanacetum vulgare

anemia
Cleome serrulata

anti-fertility
Apocynum androsaemifolium
Cnicus benedictus
Cuscuta megalocarpa
Nasturtium officinale
Panax quinquefolia
Smilacina amplexicaulis
Veratrum californicum

antiseptic
Baptisia tinctoria
Cinnamomum camphora
Geranium maculatum
Liquidambar styraciflua
Salvia officinalis

anti-smoking
Lobelia inflata

aphrodosiac
Eryngium aquaticum
Fraxinus americana
Lycopodium clavatum
Nasturtium officinale
Panax quinquefolia
Passiflora incarnata
Salix nigra
Trillium erectum

arthritis
Gaura parviflora
Glycyrrhiza lepidota
Polygonatum biflorum

asthma
Ailanthus altissima
Allium sativum
Apocynum cannabinum
Aralia racemosa
Arctium minus
Arisaema triphyllum
Asclepias syriaca
Asclepiodora viridis
Datura stramonium
Digitalis purpurea
Dioscorea villosa
Heracleum maximum
Leonurus cardiaca
Lobelia inflata
Marrubium vulgare
Opuntia tuna
Rhus glabra
Salix nigra
Smilacina amplexicaulis
Solanum carolinense
Symplocarpus foetidus
Veratrum viride
Verbascum thapsus

astringent
Baptisia tinctoria

B

backache
Aralia racemosa

bedbug
Juglans nigra

bladder
Cannabis sativa
Eryngium yuccifolium
Tephrosia virginiana
Verbesina helianthoides
Xanthium strumarium
blood poisoning
Aralia racemosa
Echinacea purpurea
Viburnum opulus
blood purifier
Alnus serrulata
Aralia spinosa
Arctium lappa
Betula lenta
Eryngium aquaticum
Populus angustifolia
Populus balsamifera
Sorbus americana
Taraxacum officinale
Verbesina helianthoides
boils
Carthamus tinctorius
Datura stramonium
Erythronium grandiflorum
Pinus edulis
Populus wislizenii
Rumex crispus
broken bones
Populus balsamifera
bronchitis
Angelica atropurpurea
Aplectrum hyemale
Arctostaphylos uva-ursi
Asclepias tuberosa
Cimicifuga racemosa
Eucalyptus globulus
Helianthus annuus
Ginkgo biloba
Juniperus virginiana
Monarda fistulosa
Sassafras albidum
Solanum carolinense
bruises, wounds
Betula papyrifera
Datura meteloides
Daucus carota
Hamamelis virginiana
Helianthus strumosus
Larix laricina
Passiflora incarnata

Plantago spp.
Populus wislizenii
Tanacetum vulgare
Taraxacum officinale
burns
Abies balsamea
Arctium lappa
Betula papyrifera
Celastrus scandens
Cupressus arizonica
Datura meteloides
Fagus grandifolia
Passiflora incarnata
Pinus strobus
Quercus alba
Rhus glabra
Sambucus canadensis
Trifolium pratense

cathartic
Juglans cinerea
childbirth
Artemisia tridentata
Caulophyllum thalictroides
Chenopodium ambrosioides
Cimicifuga americana
Cupressus arizonica
Dioscorea villosa
Fraxinus americana
Gelsemium sempervirens
Glycyrrhiza lepidota
Malva parviflora
Mentha spicata
Mitchella repens
Penstemon pallidus
Prunus serotina
Prunus virginiana
Scutellaria lateriflora
Senecio aureus
Spiraea tomentosa
Stillingia sylvatica
Trillium erectum
Ulmus rubra
Viburnum opulus
Xanthorhiza simplicissima

chills
    Monarda fistulosa
cholera
    Cornus florida
colds
    Abies balsamea
    Adiantum pedatum
    Allium sativum
    Aralia racemosa
    Brassica rapa
    Chrysanthemum parthenium
    Eupatorium perfoliatum
    Hedeoma pulegioides
    Helenium autumnale
    Ilex opaca
    Lindera benzoin
    Magnolia virginiana
    Monarda fistulosa
    Nasturtium officinale
    Nepeta cataria
    Panax quinquefolia
    Prunus serotina
    Prunus virginiana
    Salix nigra
    Salvia officinalis
    Tsuga canadensis
    Verbascum thapsus
    Verbena hastata
    Xanthorhiza simplicissima
colic
    Artemisia tridentata
    Asclepias tuberosa
    Caulophyllum thalictroides
    Chrysanthemum parthenium
    Comptonia peregrina
    Dyssodia papposa
    Gaultheria procumbens
    Heracleum maximum
    Juniperus communis
    Mentha piperita
    Pinus palustris
    Prunella vulgaris
    Ruta graveolens
    Xanthoxylum americanum
    Xanthoxylum clava-herculis
convulsions
    Hedeoma pulegioides
    Lobelia inflata
    Monotropa uniflora
    Panax quinquefolia
    Ruta graveolens
    Solanum carolinense

cramps
    Collinsonia canadensis
    Jeffersonia diphylla
croup
    Dioscorea villosa
    Polygala senega
    Verbascum thapsus
cuts, abrasions
    Abies balsamea
    Abies fraseri
    Acer rubrum
    Alnus serrulata
    Aralia racemosa
    Asclepias speciosa
    Baptisia leucophaea
    Betula papyrifera
    Chionanthus virginicus
    Geranium maculatum
    Ginkgo biloba
    Hydrastis canadensis
    Liquidambar styraciflua
    Xanthium strumarium

D

dandruff
    Euonymus americanus
depressant
    Gelsemium sempervirens
depression
    Cannabis sativa
    Chamaelirium luteum
diabetes
    Lycopus virginicus
diarrhea
    Actaea arguta
    Alnus serrulata
    Amaranthus hybridus
    Amaranthus retroflexus
    Ambrosia L. spp.
    Arctostaphylos uva-ursi
    Artemisia tridentata
    Capsella bursa-pastoris
    Chimaphila maculata
    Chionanthus virginicus
    Chrysanthemum parthenium
    Cinnamomum camphora
    Coccoloba uvifera

Comptonia peregrina
Diospyros virginiana
Dyssodia papposa
Erigeron canadensis
Fragaria virginiana
Geranium maculatum
Gillenia trifoliata
Helenium hoopesii
Helianthemum canadense
Heracleum maximum
Heuchera americana
Kallstroemia grandiflora
Kalmia latifolia
Liquidambar styraciflua
Lycopodium clavatum
Lycopus virginicus
Marrubium vulgare
Mentha spicata
Mitchella repens
Morus alba,
Opuntia tuna
Pinus palustris
Prunella vulgaris
Prunus serotina
Pteridium aquilinum
Quercus velutina
Rhus glabra
Rumex hymenosepalus
Salix alba
Salix nigra
Scutellaria lateriflora
Spiraea tomentosa
Typha laterifolia
Ulmus rubra
Vaccinium arboreum
Viburnum prunifolium

diphtheria
Eucalyptus globulus
Juglans nigra

dizziness
Panax quinquefolius

dusting powder
Lycopodium clavatum

dysentery
Ailanthus altissima
Amaranthus hybridus
Apocynum cannabinum
Berberis vulgaris
Castanea dentata
Ceanothus americanus
Cirsium flodmani
Coccoloba uvifera

Cornus florida
Diospyros virginiana
Erigeron canadensis
Eryngium aquaticum
Euphorbia maculata
Gaultheria procumbens
Geranium maculatum
Geum rivale
Lindera benzoin
Liquidambar styraciflua
Lobelia inflata
Lobelia siphilitica
Magnolia virginiana
Myrica cerifera
Opuntia spp.
Pinus strobus
Plantago spp.
Prunus virginiana
Quercus virginiana
Rubus spp.
Sassafras albidum
Serenoa serrulata
Ulmus americana
Vaccinium arboreum
Verbascum thapsus

earache
Cirsium flodmani
Melaleuca leucadendra
Verbascum thapsus

epilepsy
Ailanthus altissima
Lobelia inflata
Monotropa uniflora
Ruta graveolens
Solanum carolinense
Symplocarpus foetidus

expectorant
Arisaema triphyllum
Jeffersonia diphylla
Liquidambar styraciflua
Pinus strobus
Prunus serotina

eyes
Acer rubrum
Acer spicatum

Alnus serrulata
Aralia spinosa
Arctium lappa
Asarum canadense
Ceanothus americanus
Coptis groenlandica
Euonymus atropurpureus
Hamamelis virginiana
Hedeoma pulegioides
Hydrastis canadensis
Kallstroemia grandiflora
Kalmia latifolia
Maclura pomifera
Monotropa uniflora
Opuntia spp.
Prosopis glandulosa
Quercus alba
Quercus velutina
Quercus virginiana
Sassafras albidum
Stellaria media
Trifolium pratense

Dryopteris cristata
Eryngium aquaticum
Euonymus americanus
Euonymus atropurpureus
Eupatorium purpureum
Galium aparine
Gelsemium sempervirens
Gillenia trifoliata
Glycyrrhiza lepidota
Hepatica acutiloba
Heracleum maximum
Humulus lupulus
Ilex opaca
Kallstroemia grandiflora
Liquidambar styraciflua
Magnolia virginiana
Malva parviflora
Monarda fistulosa
Morus alba
Morus nigra
Morus rubra
Myrica cerifera
Ostrya virginiana
Oxalis violacea
Oxydendrum arboreum
Panax quinquefolius
Phytolacca americana
Podophyllum peltatum
Prunus serotina
Prunus virginiana
Rhus glabra
Salix alba
Sambucus canadensis
Sanguinaria canadensis
Thuja occidentalis
Ulmus rubra
Verbena hastata

fever blisters
Coptis groenlandica
fish poison
Echinocereus enneacanthus
Helenium amarum
Helenium autumnale
flu
Brassica rapa
Tsuga canadensis
frostbite
Fagus grandifolia
fungus infections
Juglans cinerea

facial sores
Euonymus atropurpureus
fever
Achillea millefolium
Aesculus hippocastanum
Ambrosia L. spp.
Angelica atropurpurea
Apocynum cannabinum
Aralia spinosa
Asarum canadense
Asclepiodora viridis
Baptisia tinctoria
Berberis vulgaris
Brassica rapa
Carthamus tinctorius
Cassia marilandica
Cephalanthus occidentalis
Cnicus benedictus
Coccoloba uvifera
Cornus florida
Cuscuta megalocarpa
Digitalis purpurea

gangrene
Salix nigra
gonorrhea
Ambrosia L. spp.
Arctium lappa
Asclepias syriaca
Cannabis sativa
Ceanothus americanus
Cirsium flodmani
Eryngium aquaticum
Fragaria virginiana
Ginkgo biloba
Grindelia squarrosa
Lobelia siphilitica
Opuntia tuna
Quercus alba
Rhus glabra
Rudbeckia lacinata
Typha latifolia
Xanthoxylum americanum
Xanthoxylum clava-herculis
Yucca brevifolia
gout
Angelica atropurpurea
Aralia racemosa
Arctium lappa
Betula lenta
Fragaria virginiana
Gentiana villosa
Ilex opaca
Magnolia virginiana
Menispermum canadense
Menyanthes trifoliata
Polygala senega
Saponaria officinalis
Thuja occidentalis
Veratrum viride

H

hallucinogen
Datura stramonium
Ipomoea purpurea
Mirabilis multiflora
Sanguinaria canadensis

headache
Achillea millefolium
Apocynum androsaemifolium
Artemisia tridentata
Asarum canadense
Chamaelirium luteum
Collinsonia canadensis
Cypripedium calceolus
Hedeoma pulegioides
Malva parviflora
Melaleuca leucadendra
Monarda fistulosa
Opuntia spp.
Panax quinquefolius
Prunus virginiana
Sambucus canadensis
Symplocarpus foetidus
Thalictrum fendleri
Umbellularia californica
head lice
Asimina triloba
Euonymus atropurpureus
Veratrum californicum
Veratrum viride
heart trouble
Ailanthus altissima
Apocynum androsaemifolium
Apocynum cannabinum
Asarum canadense
Asclepiodora viridis
Carthamus tinctorius
Digitalis
Heracleum maximum
Leonurus cardiaca
Nasturtium officinale
Polygala senega
Sorbus americana
Taraxacum officinale
Trillium erectum
Veratrum viride
hemorrhoid
Aesculus hippocastanum
Capsella bursa-pastoris
Collinsonia canadensis
Erigeron canadensis
Hamamelis virginiana
Passiflora incarnata
Polygonatum biflorum
Quercus alba
Stellaria media

Verbascum thapsus
Verbesina helianthoides
herpes
Liquidambar styraciflua
Veratrum viride
Xanthium strumarium
hives
Nepeta cataria
Polygala senega
Rumex crispus
hysteria
Asclepias tuberosa
Cimicifuga americana
Cinnamomum camphora
Cnicus benedictus
Lobelia inflata
Scutellaria lateriflora
Symplocarpus foetidus

Geum rivale
Gillenia trifoliata
Helenium hoopesii
Humulus lupulus
Juglans nigra
Juniperus communis
Lindera benzoin
Morus nigra
Morus rubra
Myrica cerifera
Oxalis violacea
Pinus taeda
Prunus serotina
Pteridium aquilinum
Spigelia marilandica
Symplocarpus foetidus
Tanacetum vulgare
Tephrosia virginiana
Itches
Cimicifuga racemosa
Xanthoxylum clava-herculis

I

inflammation
Humulus lupulus
insanity
Digitalis purpurea
insect bites
Cuscuta megalocarpa
Pinus edulis
Serenoa serrulata
Tanacetum vulgare
intestinal worms
Abies fraseri
Acer rubrum
Acer spicatum
Ailanthus altissima
Allium cernuum
Allium sativum
Ambrosia L. spp.
Apocynum cannabinum
Asimina
Catalpa bignonioides
Chamaelirium luteum
Chenopodium ambrosioides
Chrysanthemum parthenium
Daucus carota
Dryopteris cristata
Echinocereus enneacanthus
Eucalyptus globulus

J

jaundice
Berberis vulgaris
Chelone glabra
Cornus florida
Menyanthes trifoliata
Myrica cerifera
Podophyllum peltatum
Xanthorhiza simplicissima

K

kidney problems
Allium sativum
Apocynum androsaemifolium
Chimaphila umbellata
Cimicifuga racemosa
Diospyros virginiana
Eryngium aquaticum
Eryngium yuccifolium
Fragaria virginiana

Hydrangea arborescens
Juniperus communis
Marrubium vulgare
Nasturtium officinale
Picea mariana
Pinus palustris
Populus balsamifera
Rudbeckia laciniata
Sassafras albidum
Senecio aureus
Tiarella corcifolia
Ulmus americana

L

laryngitis
Pinus edulis
laxative
Actaea arguta
Apocynum androsaemifolium
Apocynum cannabinum
Asclepias syriaca
Baptisia tinctoria
Brassica rapa
Carthamus tinctorius
Cassia marilandica
Catalpa bignonioides
Cephalanthus occidentalis
Chelone glabra
Chenopodium album
Chrysanthemum parthenium
Cuscuta megalocarpa
Erythrina herbacea
Euonymus americanus
Euonymus atropurpureus
Eupatorium perfoliatum
Euphorbia maculata
Gillenia trifoliata
Hydrangea arborescens
Ilex opaca
Ilex vomitoria
Ipomoea purpurea
Juglans nigra
Larix laricina
Magnolia virginiana
Marrubium vulgare
Menispermum canadense
Menyanthes trifoliata

Morus alba
Morus rubra
Nasturtium officinale
Ostrya virginiana
Pinus strobus
Pinus taeda
Plantago spp.
Podophyllum peltatum
Polygala senega
Polygonatum biflorum
Quercus velutina
Rhamnus purshiana
Rumex crispus
Rumex obtusifolius
Salvia officinalis
Stillingia sylvatica
Taraxacum officinale
Tephrosia virginiana
Ulmus rubra
Veronicastrum
Viola canadensis
Viola pedata
liver problems
Cnicus benedictus
Cornus florida
Dioscorea villosa
Eryngium yuccifolium
Euonymus atropurpureus
Grindelia squarrosa
Hepatica acutiloba
Hydrastis canadensis
Podophyllum peltatum
Stillingia sylvatica
Taraxacum officinale
Trifolium pratense
lumbago
Salix nigra
lung disease
Grindelia squarrosa

malaria
Alnus serrulata
Aristolochia serpentaria
Chionanthus virginicus
Cimicifuga racemosa
Cornus florida

Eupatorium perfoliatum
Gutierrezia sarothrae
Magnolia virginiana
Ostrya virginiana
Prunus virginiana
Spigelia marilandica
Trilisa odoratissima
Verbascum thapsus
Viburnum nudum

measles
Asclepias speciosa
Carthamus tinctorius
Prunus serotina
Prunus virginiana

menstrual problems
Adiantum capillus-veneris
Amaranthus hybridus
Amaranthus retroflexus
Angelica atropurpurea
Arctium minus
Artemisia tridentata
Capsella bursa-pastoris
Carthamus tinctorius
Caulophyllum thalictroides
Celastrus scandens
Chenopodium ambrosioides
Chrysanthemum parthenium
Daucus carota
Gaultheria procumbens
Geum rivale
Glycyrrhiza lepidota
Hedeoma pulegioides
Juniperus communis
Juniperus virginiana
Malva parviflora
Marrubium vulgare
Nepeta cataria
Pinus palustris
Polygonum hydropiper
Rudbeckia laciniata
Ruta graveolens
Salix alba
Salsola kali
Scutellaria lateriflora
Stillingia sylvatica
Symplocarpus foetidus
Tanacetum vulgare
Taxus brevifolia

miscarriage
Chamaelirium luteum

moles
Asclepias syriaca

mouth sores
Chionanthus virginicus
Cornus florida
Myrica cerifera
Vicia faba
Xanthorhiza simplicissima
Xanthoxylum americanum

muscular pain, spasms
Caulophyllum thalictroides
Cinnamomum camphora
Cornus florida
Dioscorea villosa
Eryngium yuccifolium
Gaura parviflora
Hamamelis virginiana
Hedeoma pulegioides
Jeffersonia diphylla
Mentha piperita
Pinus edulis
Pinus strobus
Prunus serotina
Tephrosia virginiana
Viburnum prunifolium
Xanthoxylum clava-herculis

narcotic
Datura meteloides

neck pain
Asclepiodora viridis

nervous conditions
Asarum canadense
Cannabis sativa
Celastrus scandens
Chimaphila maculata
Cimicifuga racemosa
Cinnamomum camphora
Cypripedium calceolus
Gentiana villosa
Ginkgo biloba
Nepeta cataria
Panax quinquefolius
Quercus velutina
Senecio aureus
Solanum carolinense
Tanacetum vulgare

neuralgia
Aconitum columbianum

Actaea arguta
Aesculus hippocastanum
Cinnamomum camphora
Digitalis purpurea
Eryngium aquaticum
Mentha spicata
Ruta graveolens
nosebleed
Capsella bursa-pastoris
Eryngium aquaticum
nose, throat inflammations
Eucalyptus globulus

pain reliever
Cypripedium calceolus
Gaultheria procumbens
Gelsemium sempervirens
Monotropa uniflora
Prunus serotina
Solanum carolinense
pleurisy
Cephalanthus occidentalis
Gelsemium sempervirens
Polygala senega
pneumonia
Apocynum cannabinum
Aristolochia serpentaria
Corallorhiza maculata
Grindelia squarrosa
Hedeoma pulegioides
Lobelia inflata
Malva parviflora
Polygala senega
Vicia faba
poisoning
Aristolochia serpentaria
Artemisia tridentata
Eryngium aquaticum
pulmonary problems
Erigeron canadensis
Helenium hoopesii

rabies
Echinacea purpurea

Leonurus cardiaca
Scutellaria lateriflora
rat poison
Erythrina herbacea
respiratory problems
Abies fraseri
Adiantum capillus-veneris
Adiantum pedatum
Alnus serrulata
Arctium minus
Capsella bursa-pastoris
Ceanothus americanus
Cimicifuga americana
Cnicus benedictus
Collinsonia canadensis
Datura meteloides
Dioscorea villosa
Dryopteris cristata
Eryngium yuccifolium
Eucalyptus globulus
Gelsemium sempervirens
Ginkgo biloba
Glycyrrhiza lepidota
Helianthus annuus
Helianthus strumosus
Lobelia siphilitica
Magnolia virginiana
Melaleuca leucadendra
Nepeta cataria
Picea rubens
Pinus taeda
Polygala senega
Populus balsamifera
Prunus virginiana
Quercus alba
Sanguinaria canadensis
Sassafras albidum
Serenoa serrulata
Stellaria pubera
Stillingia sylvatica
Symplocarpus foetidus
Tiarella cordifolia
Ulmus rubra
Verbena hastata
Viola pedata
Xanthoxylum clava-herculis
rheumatism
Actaea arguta
Aesculus hippocastanum
Aletris farinosa
Angelica atropurpurea
Arctium lappa

Arctium minus
Arisaema triphyllum
Artemisia tridentata
Asclepias speciosa
Betula lenta
Caulophyllum thalictroides
Chimaphila maculata
Chimaphila umbellata
Cimicifuga americana
Cimicifuga racemosa
Cinnamomum camphora
Comptonia peregrina
Dioscorea villosa
Erodium cicutarium
Eryngium yuccifolium
Gaultheria procumbens
Gentiana villosa
Gillenia trifoliata
Glycyrrhiza lepidota
Grindelia squarrosa
Gutierrezia sarothrae
Helenium hoopesii
Helianthus annuus
Heracleum maximum
Humulus lupulus
Ilex opaca
Jeffersonia diphylla
Juniperus virginiana
Larix laricina
Magnolia virginiana
Menispermum canadense
Mentha spicata
Menyanthes trifoliata
Opuntia tuna
Panax quinquefolius
Picea mariana
Picea rubens
Pinus strobus
Polygala senega
Polygonatum biflorum
Populus balsamifera
Quercus alba
Quercus velutina
Robinia neo-mexicana
Ruta graveolens
Sambucus canadensis
Sanguinaria canadensis
Saponaria officinalis
Symplocarpus foetidus
Thuja occidentalis
Umbellularia californica
Veratrum viride

Xanthoxylum americanum
Xanthoxylum clava-herculis
rib pain
Asclepiodora viridis
ringworm
Asclepias speciosa
Cupressus arizonica
Morus rubra
Rumex crispus
Symplocarpus foetidus

scabies
Liquidambar styraciflua
Melaleuca leucadendra
scarlet fever
Baptisia leucophaea
Baptisia tinctoria
Jeffersonia diphylla
scurvy
Menyanthes trifoliata
Myrica cerifera
Populus balsamifera
Sorbus americana
Stellaria pubera
Thuja occidentalis
Viburnum opulus
sedative
Aletris farinosa
Castanea dentata
Ceanothus americanus
Corallorhiza maculata
Cypripedium calceolus
Datura stramonium
Humulus lupulus
Lactuca scariola
Lycopus virginicus
Prunus virginiana
Ruta graveolens
Scutellaria lateriflora
Serenoa serrulata
Solanum carolinense
Trifolium pratense
skin problems
Achillea millefolium
Alnus serrulata
Ambrosia L. spp.

Arctium lappa
Arctostaphylos uva-ursi
Betula lenta
Carthamus tinctoris
Catalpa bignonioides
Chimaphila maculata
Chionanthus virginicus
Cimicifuga americana
Cupressus arizonica
Dicentra cucullaria
Echinacea purpurea
Euonymus americanus
Fagus grandifolia
Grindelia squarrosa
Hamamelis virginiana
Helianthemum canadensis
Heuchera americana
Juniperus virginiana
Kalmia latifolia
Malva parviflora
Melaleuca leucadendra
Menispermum canadense
Menyanthes trifoliata
Monarda fistulosa
Passiflora incarnata
Phytolacca americana
Pinus strobus
Pinus taeda
Polygonatum biflorum
Prosopis glandulosa
Rhus glabra
Rumex crispus
Rumex obtusifolius
Salvia officinalis
Sambucus canadensis
Sanguinaria canadensis
Serenoa serrulata
Stellaria media
Symplocarpus foetidus
Trillium erectum
Trifolium pratense
Ulmus americana
Verbascum thapsus
Viola canadensis
Xanthium strumarium

sleep aid
Cypripedium calceolus

smallpox
Aristolochia serpentaria
Grindelia squarrosa

snakebite
Allium sativum

Aralia spinosa
Asclepias speciosa
Cimicifuga americana
Echinacea purpurea
Eryngium yuccifolium
Erythronium grandiflorum
Fraxinus americana
Gutierrezia sarothrae
Juniperus communis
Penstemon pallidus
Polygala senega
Populus balsamifera
Serenoa serrulata

sores
Abies balsamea
Aesculus hippocastanum
Alnus serrulata
Aralia racemosa
Arctium lappa
Artemisia tridentata
Asclepias speciosa
Asclepias tuberosa
Baptisia tinctoria
Cassia marilandica
Caulophyllum thalictroides
Ceanothus americanus
Cimicifuga racemosa
Datura meteloides
Diospyros virginiana
Erigeron canadensis
Fraxinus americana
Geranium maculatum
Helianthemum canadense
Heuchera americana
Hydrastis canadensis
Jeffersonia diphylla
Kallstroemia grandiflora
Lactuca scariola
Mentha piperita
Mentha spicata
Monarda fistulosa
Pinus edulis
Polygonum hydropiper
Prosopis glandulosa
Prunella vulgaris
Prunus virginiana
Quercus alba
Rhus glabra
Rumex hymenosepalus
Salvia officinalis
Sambucus canadensis
Sanguinaria canadensis

Symplocarpus foetidus
Vaccinium arboreum
Verbascum thapsus
Xanthoxylum americanum

spleen

Taraxacum officinale

stimulant

Abies fraseri
Achillea millefolium
Acorus calamus
Adiantum pedatum
Aralia spinosa
Asarum canadense
Baptisia leucophaea
Ceanothus americanus
Cinnamomum camphora
Eupatorium purpureum
Hedeoma pulegioides
Juniperus virginiana
Leonurus cardiaca
Lindera benzoin
Mentha piperita
Mentha spicata
Panax quinquefolius
Pinus taeda
Tephrosia virginiana
Xanthoxylum clava-herculis

stomach problems

Achillea millefolium
Acorus calamus
Ailanthus altissima
Aletris farinosa
Angelica atropurpurea
Apocynum cannabinum
Arctium minus
Arctostaphylos uva-ursi
Arisaema triphyllum
Artemisia tridentata
Asarum canadense
Asclepias syriaca
Berberis vulgaris
Brassica rapa
Caulophyllum thalictroides
Chenopodium album
Chimaphila umbellata
Chrysanthemum parthenium
Collinsonia canadensis
Coptis groenlandica
Cupressus arizonica
Dioscorea villosa
Dyssodia papposa
Euonymus atropurpureus

Franseria tenuifolia
Gaultheria procumbens
Gelsemium sempervirens
Gentiana villosa
Geum rivale
Gillenia trifoliata
Ginkgo biloba
Glycyrrhiza lepidota
Grindelia squarrosa
Gutierrezia sarothrae
Helenium hoopesii
Heracleum maximum
Hydrastis canadensis
Juniperus communis
Kallstroemia grandiflora
Larix laricina
Mentha piperita
Mentha spicata
Menyanthes trifoliata
Mirabilis multiflora
Monarda fistulosa
Nepeta cataria
Ostrya virginiana
Picea mariana
Picea rubens
Populus balsamifera
Prosopis glandulosa
Prunella vulgaris
Prunus serotina
Prunus virginiana
Pteridium aquilinum
Ruta graveolens
Salix nigra
Salvia officinalis
Sassafras albidum
Serenoa serrulata
Spigelia marilandica
Tanacetum vulgare
Taraxacum officinale
Trifolium pratense
Umbellularia californica
Veratrum viride
Verbena hastata
Verbesina helianthoides
Xanthorhiza simplicissima
Xanthoxylum clava-herculis

sunburn

Verbascum thapsus

swellings

Asclepias speciosa
Celastrus scandens
Cleome serrulata

Gaultheria procumbens
Geranium maculatum
Nepeta cataria
Opuntia spp.
Ostrya virginiana
Oxydendrum arboreum
Pinus strobus
Tsuga canadensis

syphilis

Alnus serrulata
Arctium lappa
Ceanothus americanus
Chimaphila maculata
Echinacea purpurea
Euonymus atropurpureus
Helianthemum canadense
Jeffersonia diphylla
Juglans nigra
Kalmia latifolia
Lobelia siphilitica
Menispermum canadense
Pinus edulis
Podophyllum peltatum
Saponaria officinalis
Stillingia sylvatica
Tephrosia virginiana

Chimaphila umbellata
Dicentra cucullaria
Eupatorium purpureum
Gentiana villosa
Gillenia trifoliata
Hydrangea arborescens
Hydrastis canadensis
Ilex vomitoria
Lactuca scariola
Larix laricina
Leonurus cardiaca
Magnolia virginiana
Marrubium vulgare
Menispermum canadense
Ostrya virginiana
Oxalis violacea
Oxydendrum arboreum
Panax quinquefolius
Plantago spp.
Quercus velutina
Rhamnus purshiana
Salix alba
Salvia officinalis
Sambucus canadensis
Sanguinaria canadensis
Stellaria pubera
Taraxacum officinale
Tephrosia virginiana
Ulmus americana
Viburnum nudum
Viburnum prunifolium
Xanthoxylum clava-herculis

tuberculosis

Achillea millefolium
Arisaema triphyllum
Asclepias speciosa
Cuscuta megalocarpa
Eucalyptus globulus
Ilex opaca
Lycopus virginicus
Nasturtium officinale
Pinus palustris
Prunus serotina
Prunus virginiana
Quercus velutina
Stellaria pubera
Xanthium strumarium

tumors

Pinus palustris
Podophyllum peltatum

typhoid

Baptisia leucophaea

tetanus

Cannabis sativa
Solanum carolinense

throat problems

Chionanthus virginicus
Xanthorhiza simplicissima
Xanthoxylum clava-herculis

tonic

Acer rubrum
Achillea millefolium
Acorus calamus
Aesculus hippocastanum
Aletris farinosa
Apocynum androsaemifolium
Castanea dentata
Cephalanthus occidentalis
Chelone glabra
Chimaphila maculata

typhus
- Aristolochia serpentaria
- Baptisia tinctoria
- Chimaphila umbellata
- Eupatorium purpureum

ulcer
- Baptisia tinctoria
- Chimaphila maculata
- Rumex obtusifolius
- Salix nigra
- Spiraea tomentosa
- Xanthoxylum americanum
- Xanthoxylum clava-herculis

V

venereal disease
- Caulophyllum thalictroides
- Celastrus scandens
- Cephalanthus occidentalis
- Dicentra cucullaria
- Euonymus americanus
- Rumex obtusifolius

W

warts
- Asclepias syriaca
- Euphorbia maculata
- Salvia officinalis
- Thuja occidentalis

weakness
- Asclepias tuberosa
- Comptonia peregrina
- Senecio aureus

whooping cough
- Castanea dentata
- Lobelia inflata
- Trifolium pratense

worms
- Artemisia tridentata
- Castanea dentata
- Chelone glabra
- Corallorhiza maculata
- Cornus florida
- Eupatorium perfoliatum
- Ginkgo biloba
- Ilex opaca
- Juglans cinerea
- Juglans nigra
- Melaleuca leucadendra
- Menyanthes trifoliata
- Pinus palustris
- Prunus virginiana
- Salvia officinalis
- Tephrosia virginiana
- Typha latifolia

wounds
- Aristolochia serpentaria
- Artemisia tridentata
- Baptisia tinctoria
- Chionanthus virginicus
- Datura stramonium
- Geranium maculatum
- Juniperus communis
- Liquidambar styraciflua
- Panax quinquefolius
- Phytolacca americana
- Picea mariana
- Pinus palustris
- Pinus strobus
- Salvia officinalis
- Typha latifolia
- Ulmus rubra
- Veratrum viride
- Xanthoxylum americanum

yellow fever
- Cimicifuga racemosa